About the author:

Ralf R. Rompard M.D. is a General Practitioner licensed in Hong Kong and in England.

THROUGH THE GREAT WALL

A Western Acupuncture Doctor in the People's Republic of China

Ralf Robert Rompard

Book Guild Publishing

First published in Great Britain in 2015 by
The Book Guild Ltd
9 Priory Business Park
Wistow Road
Kibworth
Leics LE8 0RX
Email: info@bookguild.co.uk
Freephone: 0800 999 2982
Web: www.bookguild.co.uk
Twitter: @bookguild

Typesetting in Garamond by
YHT Ltd, London

Printed and bound in Great Britain by
CPI Group (UK) Ltd, Croydon, CR0 4YY

A catalogue record for this book is available from
The British Library.

ISBN 978 1 910508 76 3

Contents

OH, East is East, and West is West, and never the twain shall meet,
Till Earth and Sky stand presently at God's great Judgment Seat;
But there is neither East nor West, Border, nor Breed, nor Birth,
When two strong men stand face to face, tho' they come from the ends
of the earth!

(Rudyard Kipling, *The Ballad of East and West*)

I

Into the Middle Kingdom

The flight from Geneva to Beijing was scheduled to take eighteen hours. I had booked a window seat in the front part of the plane and was enjoying Swissair service. Stopovers were planned in Athens, Dubai, Delhi and Bangkok to take on fuel. During these, passengers could avail themselves of an opportunity to stretch their legs. On board were several European medical men and women on their way to China, there to study acupuncture at first hand. We had taken the opportunity of getting to know one another superficially in the transit lounges, but in this atmosphere there was no real opportunity to get beyond the murmured names. Anyway, I now knew that behind me in the plane there were other doctors who had the same intentions as me.

I had brought with me a number of things to read. In the plane's cabin I had found a copy of the Zurich newspaper *Neue Zürcher Zeitung*. That should be enough to keep me occupied until we landed in Beijing. But there was other reading matter packed away in my suitcase: a book on the analysis of Chinese pictograms by Leon Wieger together with a translation of the Dao De Jing by the German clergyman Richard Wilhelm, another book published by Rowohlt Publishers on Mao Tse-tung and the 'New China', as well as new Chinese publications on medicine and acupuncture. It was for this reason that my suitcase weighed almost 10 kilos more than was allowed. However, I had been lucky not to be asked to pay an extra fee for this as a passenger in the tourist class. The Swissair personnel knew that I was on a trip to Beijing with other doctors.

Around noon on the second day of our flight we flew over the snow-covered Himalayas, and after the Chinese border lay behind us it was clear how intensively cultivated the country below us was. Everywhere there were long, straight canals which now glittered in the noonday sun. A few of these flowed into mirror-like lake complexes. Square rice fields stretched before us to the bluish-brown horizon. They were like an immense patchwork carpet thrown out to cover the land, a strong testament to the achievement of a thousand years of agricultural planning and irrigation – China's stomach.

I was impressed by the new era of Chinese politics. I had completed a number of Chinese language courses at the German Society for East Asian Studies, where the majority of our tutors and professors were themselves Chinese and also fierce Maoists. They had done much to motivate my interest in Chinese Communism. In a text publication I had once written to the effect that Mao Tse-tung was not only and merely a hope for the Middle Kingdom, but also a hope for the western world. Here is an excerpt:

'Mao the Great Chairman of the Chinese Communist Party is fond of expressing his insights in pithy sentences. One of these is: "Let a hundred flowers bloom; let a hundred schools of thought compete with one another." '

My commentary at the time was as follows:

'This shows a tolerance, which gets to grips with real problems and also demonstrates a more just recognition of things than the rigid, positivistic rationalism of the West. As far as this is concerned, Mao's attitude is not a mere "ideology", which many Western critics would have us believe. On the contrary, it is based on what we could call a thoroughly scientific critical awareness. In the meantime we have this to thank for the renaissance of China's traditional medicine and, as a result, numerous patients in the West could be cured, while their own so-called "scientific" medicine had failed to help them.'

At the time of writing this, I didn't yet know that Mao's 'hundred flowers' metaphor was not to be understood as marking the beginning of freedom of thought in politics, but rather, this 'blooming of flowers' was merely a means of exposing the development of liberal streams of thought under his sway in order to nip these developments in the bud and put their proponents in 'educational' camps, there to brutally subject them to torture or to condemn them to death without the right to be heard by a just body of law.

I was fascinated by Mao, especially since every book published on acupuncture and traditional medicine in China included a preface written in his own spidery scrawl. There was practically no work of this kind from the mainland which did not enthusiastically acknowledge his commitment to maintaining the principles of Chinese traditional medicine. Was it possible, then, to doubt all this? Recognising this, I went on in my text to quote Mao further:

'We are in a position to study what we don't understand for the time being. We will know not only how to destroy the old world, but will also know how to build the new.'

A new world such as this, I felt, was something urgently needed in the West as well, and it called to mind the following passage which had appeared in Gregorio Bermann's book *Social Psychiatry in China*:

'The most outstanding fact in Chinese psychiatry is the low number of mentally sick people in the country.'

Was this really true?

I had travelled in China for the first time three years previously, but my impressions gained now were to revise my earlier unalloyed enthusiasm. Why, I asked myself, did hundreds of thousands of refugees stream across China's border each year to find asylum in Hong Kong? This was always coupled with the danger of being caught by Red Army soldiers and shot on the spot. Wasn't there a parallel here with the East–West border that existed in Germany at that time? People were willing to risk their lives fleeing from the German Democratic Republic either over the infamous wall in Berlin or along the so-called green border where they were exposed to automatic, self-releasing gunfire batteries or snipers. And all this to gain freedom. Tears came into his eyes as a Chinese doctor who had studied western medicine in Guangzhou (Canton) told me, for example, of how he and his wife had swum the South China Sea naked from the Chinese mainland in shark-infested water that was studded with sharp coral, to freedom in Hong Kong. They were young and both of them had trained hard before their adventure and for this reason had overcome their ordeal. Others had either been torn apart by sharks or succumbed to a hail of bullets. Death was more desirable than life in a communist hell. Apparently something there was seriously wrong.

In these days, I was also sickened by western civilisation. I found the peevish criticism of the current German political relations indulged in by intellectuals quite nauseating. German writers publishing books by guess-work, yet knowing nothing of the real world outside them, simply bored me to death. Then there were the small-minded philistines from so-called higher circles, stinking of synthetic perfume to be found at symphony concerts and at opera and theatrical performances whom I found repellent. And as for the growing vulgarity and violence associated with sport – football, for example – which had in the meantime become an epidemic, one could only speak of this as being rife with horror. Moreover, I felt disappointed with the prevailing attitudes of the majority of my colleagues in medicine. So many of them were puffed up with swank or consumed by the desire for money and possessions. So for these reasons I decided to keep a diary of my everyday experiences as an acupuncture student and practising physician while in China. In addition, I wanted to note down marginal experiences too. These, I felt, would furnish a refreshing contrast to life in Europe.

To pass the time while aboard the aircraft, I drew one or two Chinese characters on the menu. I jotted down all I could see from the window: the sky, the earth, mountains, clouds, water, the sun, rice and rice fields, canals, medicine, and the pictograph for China…

My neighbour leaned over towards me. 'You can write Chinese?'

Like me, he had boarded the plane in Geneva, and he had sat next to me since stopping over in Dubai. He was on his way to China to study Chinese medicine, too. More exactly, he was out to learn what we call 'acupuncture'.

'It helps me to concentrate,' I replied.

'But isn't it a rather abstruse or – forgive me – even an idiotic language,' he said, at the same time introducing himself as Dr Haubensack, surgeon and consultant from Nancy in France. 'It has no logic!'

'Well, it's based on the logic of pictorial representation,' I said.

'What does that mean? They don't help us much, these pictures, do they?' he objected. 'The world today runs on the lines of a logic created by western language.'

'Sometimes pictures get us nearer to reality than words and letters.'

'You think so?'

'Perhaps we can bore through the Great Wall with Chinese characters to get an idea of what's behind it and so understand the Chinese better.'

The surgeon thought I was joking. 'Odd, but interesting nevertheless,' he countered politely. 'I guess we'll learn quite a bit about these things in the coming months. One of my hobbies is history, by the way. I've taken the trouble to prepare myself in this direction with a few books on Far Eastern history and one or two more recent works in the way of acquainting myself with Chinese medicine.'

He was probably about fifty or so, wore a small blond moustache, had full, loose hair and was dressed in an elegant tailored suit. There was certain loftiness in his expression, the eyes and manner revealing determination, but humour was there too.

'Look down there at that irrigation system, the artificial waterways,' I said. He leaned across to get a better view of the scenery below us.

'I've read about them,' he said. 'They go back to an ancient Chinese emperor called Yu who secured China's rural fertility by installing artificial waterways, with the result that the annual flooding was stopped. It guaranteed the population of that time – probably hundreds of thousands, but perhaps a million or so – sufficient food to live on.'

Inspired by the gliding landscape below, he went on: 'Another emperor named Huang Di deserves to be remembered for his services to his subjects in the matter of health – including acupuncture. In this, he worked together with a third emperor called Shen Nung who, as a man versed in farming, studied the attributes of health-promoting plants and placed them into various categories. While about official business, he was ever busy chewing leaves, herbs and roots and was the first to categorise them.'

I added that he was the first to give the Chinese a book on healing herbs. Named after him, it was entitled *The Root and Herb Classic by Shen Nung.*

'I see you've been doing your homework,' my neighbour said.

We were quiet for a while and then my neighbour, who, as a Frenchman, had indulged himself in several glasses of red wine at lunch, fell asleep. He began to snore loudly.

While I watched the countryside below pass by slowly under the influence of the advancing evening, the mountains, the lakes and the canals were gradually losing their contours in mist. I began to think about the value nations placed on culture and what role this played in their inhabitants' private lives. Sometimes culture may well force us into artificial roles which, on occasion, can lead us to protest, since it produces a straightjacket for the individual. On the other hand, it can give us a protective shield under which we find our daily bread, and not only that, but also an opportunity to understand nature, to learn about minerals, plant life, animals and human beings. Culture and nature, a team in double harness at work in our history and having two quite different faces. Yet I would have liked to create one vision from both features.

Some of our great cultures had been able more fully than others to disclose nature – that which we so familiarly call 'Mother Nature' in European tradition. In this, I felt, ancient China had shown itself to be a past master. Why was this so?

This question had been gnawing at me for years and was one of the reasons I was aboard this plane today on the way to Beijing. For medical professionals, culture is of particular importance. Our profession has not only come about from knowledge of the ways of nature, it has also issued from the culture in which it finds itself. Healing is the application of nature. At the same time, healing is one of the most basic natural processes in cultural achievement. Culture means upholding tradition and thus implies responsibility, the need to learn for a lifetime and to adapt to norms and, simultaneously, it implies a critical attitude, one which enquires about the why and how of that which has come down to us. It also implies a critical stance towards outdated thinking habits in order to better understand our world and the people in it. In our own case, it means setting up a good system of healing, and being able to constantly adjust this to what is required of us. That, in so many words, is what constitutes the 'art of medical practice'.

Today, this indigenous skill has fallen victim to the tricks and dodges of opportunistic politicians and, egged on by these, their superficial bureaucrats have followed suit to destroy the art of healing. This has happened not only in Europe, but also in the rest of the western world. It could well be that the organisers of this situation see themselves as winners by having substituted a sterile system of professional fees and charges in the place of medical creativity. But for the time being they are working against the natural, ever-renewable spring active in the art of healing. The possibility of a regeneration of the art of healing fills them with fear, and for the moment a treacherous silence reigns. However, the living source at the basis of medicine will leave them with no peace. Many European doctors want to return at last to the roots of their cherished profession.

My neighbour had woken up in the meantime. He blinked in my direction. It seemed as though he wanted to pursue our conversation again. Discreetly, I continued my thoughts and said, 'Life is short and art is long.'

'I beg your pardon . . . ?'

'That's what our great founding forefather, Hippocrates, wrote,' I said. 'I'm sure you're acquainted with the aphorism! It contains an admonishing "Thank your professional forerunners. Honour your teachers on whose shoulders you stand and without whom you would not know what you know and be what you are." '

'That's right,' the Frenchman said dryly. 'We keep to that every day – why, then, all the talk about it?' He ordered a coffee and took up the thread again. 'I wonder, do you think the ancient Chinese had a kind of Hippocratic Oath of their own? Did they also have an ethical guideline in their professional activity?'

Although the text had hung in my study for years, I had forgotten the actual wording.

My colleague then went on to quote the following oath in German:

'I swear by Apollo the physician, by Asklepios, by Hygieia and Panakeia and by all the gods and goddesses here as my witnesses, that I will carry out, according to my ability and judgement, this oath and this indenture. To hold my teacher in this art equal to my own parents; to make him partner in my livelihood; when he is in need of money to share mine with him; to consider his family as my own brothers, and to teach them this art, if they want to learn it, without fee or indenture; to impart instruction, written, oral and practical to my own sons, the sons of my teacher, and to indentured pupils who have taken the physician's oath, but to nobody else. I will use treatment to help the sick according to my ability and judgement, but never with a view to injury and wrong-doing. Neither will I administer a poison to anybody when asked to do so, nor will I suggest such a course etc. . . . Now if I carry out this oath, and break it not, may I gain for ever reputation among all men for my life and for my art; but if I transgress it and forswear myself, may the opposite befall me.'

His German was almost without an accent and this astonished me.

'I was born in Strasbourg,' he said. 'That's to say, I'm not only a Frenchman, but an Alsatian. One of my grandmothers and one of my grandfathers came from Germany, one from Baden and the other from the Rhine area. At home we spoke German for the most part. At school, though, and later at university, I was obliged to speak French. So I grew up with the two languages. Actually, I speak three languages. Alsatian is a dialect I speak at home, and that ought to count, too! Anyway, let's get back to our theme: was there such a thing as a written professional code in ancient China?'

'Indeed there was. In ancient China there was an ethical code governing the activities of those wishing to practise Chen-chiu – that is to say, needle and moxa therapy. The text is to be found in the book *Ling-Shu Jing*. Here, the Emperor Huang Di is speaking to an aspiring medical student, Lee-Kung:

'"Only if a doctor aspires to work for the welfare of others and if he is reliable and does not think of personal enrichment, should he be instructed in the art of needle treatment. If you are interested in a charitable activity, why don't you give me a ceremonial promise?"

'Lee Kung goes away and over the next three days prepares himself. He eats no meat, drinks no alcohol and renounces all sexual contact. On the fourth day, the Emperor accompanies him to a special room in the palace where he is sworn in. The emperor takes a knife and inflicts a deep wound on the student's upper arm, allowing the blood to flow freely from the injury. He then takes some of the blood and coats the young man's lips with it. Then he says:

'"From noon on today you are a privileged doctor and shall be initiated into the secrets of Chen-chiu. You are to study further and your conduct shall be beyond impeachment. If this should not be so, and you violate this promise, know that you will do great damage to your profession. The consequences for you of such a violation will be that you will be pursued by personal misfortune."

'The young man assures the Emperor of his dependability, at which Huang Di then passes the textbook on the classical techniques of Chen-chiu to the doctor and at the same time announces that he will teach him personally.'

Dr Haubensack, my neighbour, was surprised. 'Educated Chinese, as represented by their emperor, have indeed demanded a code of ethical behaviour similar to that prescribed by the ancient Greeks and later adopted by Europeans?' he asked. 'But is there still such a code in operation today, I wonder? Can we still find the harmony which was once a Chinese tradition embodying nature and culture in the ethics of today's rulers and physicians?'

'We'll know all about that in a few weeks, I suppose.'

'I hope so!'

The red of an evening sun dimmed behind the western mountain ranges. One peak we could see quite clearly against the horizon towering majestically above the plain is called Kun-Lun. This also happens to be the name of a structure in Chinese acupuncture which lies above the heel bone at the side of the human foot. When this spot is appropriately punctured with a needle, it is effective against kidney disease, sciatica, migraine, cervical spasms and pain in the back. Thus, ancient Chinese medicine was inseparably bound up with what we call nature. For those privileged to be initiated into its secrets, it was soon understood that they were being introduced to a whole. This wholeness included the earth, the moon, the sun and the heavens, with man himself occupying a place at the centre of things. Wind and water, heat and cold, dryness and fire, the stars, the whole world and the cosmos are reflected even today in the classical Chinese characters which, as in antiquity, are still essential for a proper understanding of ancient China and its medicine.

Now the canals below going back thousands of years began to shimmer softly in a mixture of turquoise and violet haze which was slowly swallowing up the earth as the weak red sun sank behind the horizon. I leaned back in my seat and stretched my legs. The last European meal was served. The Occident was behind us for good.

On landing in Beijing we were greeted at the airport by hundreds of red flags flapping in the wind. Uniformed troops were everywhere. Soldiers of the National Liberation Army with the blood-red star on their green caps stood lined up stiffly to attention as though awaiting the arrival of an international dignitary. Groups of girl ballet dancers with blue feather skirts hopped and skipped in picturesque Chinese traditional costumes, themselves arranged, like the soldiers, in strict order, and sang with high falsetto voices while waving coloured pennants to and fro in the evening under glaring floodlights. A band played slow march music. I recognised the melody as 'Dong Fan Hong' – 'The East is Red'. It was the Chinese national anthem.

'So much honour?' my neighbour enquired.

'I don't think it's for us; doctors are not so important in communist China,' I replied.

We found out soon enough that the reception was for a state guest who had flown with us in first class without anyone knowing about it. He and his associates had enjoyed special privileges on board. They were politicians accompanying the President of Guyana, in South America, who had come to attend governmental talks in the capital.

'Are politics more important in China than medicine?' my colleague asked.

'That's what we have to assume,' I replied. 'But isn't that the case everywhere?'

'I guess so,' the Frenchman replied.

The privileged passengers were the first to disembark. All of them were greeted by a row of about ten functionaries, all dressed in the same mousy grey 'Mao-look' outfits. They stood on a red carpet and welcomed their guests with a handshake. The Great Chairman, Mao, had succumbed to Parkinson's disease shortly after my last visit to the People's Republic. For years, communist China had called an army of western neurologists and surgeons to consultations in Beijing in an attempt to find a cure for Mao's kind of disorder. Either Chinese medicine had failed to relieve him of his complaint or Mao himself only wanted to avail himself of western medicine. This man who had for years insisted that his subjects adhere strictly to Chinese medical treatment, and who had with much propaganda even exported it into the West, wished only to be treated by western medicine himself, because he felt it to be far superior to his native curative methods – like many of his countrymen, by the way. For high-ranking politicians there, as in every communist state, only the best is good enough, and so not much is left over for the people. I could not make out whether the lanky, broad-shouldered figure among the reception committee was in fact Hua Guo-Feng, the new party leader whom I had seen in photographs, with his fleshy, round face shining greasily in the artificial light.

We were obliged to wait until the political formalities were at an end and the crowd had disappeared before we could descend to the runway. It was a kind of agony waiting there until everything was completely over. After going through passport and customs formalities and finally luggage control, we were formally received by the officials in charge of our respective diplomatic mission. A woman council member for cultural affairs from the German embassy greeted me, and then we were securely packed into black diplomatic corps saloon cars and driven to our hotels.

It was still quite warm there in the evening – much warmer than when we took off in Switzerland. A fresh wind swept over from Mongolia in the north, making the red communist flags flutter. Green-uniformed soldiers belonging to the so-called National Liberation Army controlled the streets, which were filled with wave upon wave of cyclists surging endlessly along, ringing their bells which, from the distance, sounded like the chirping of millions of cicadas. The air was full, too, of the unrhythmical, staccato honking of coaches and the rattle and grind of the few old cars and heaving, dusty trucks. Individuals walking alone were rarely seen. Here, people en masse dictated the scene, especially on the streets of Beijing. We had finally arrived. Mainland China's capital had opened its doors to us.

China – a Baptism

Today was our second day in the Chinese metropolis. We were staying at the Beijing Hotel. However, not in the well-appointed, modern wing of the hotel in which I was privileged to be accommodated on my last visit three years ago, but in another, rather run-down part of the old building. This was probably due to the fact that we had been invited as visitors of the government – that is, as 'guests' of the country. In other words, whereas three years ago I was obliged to pay for my lodging out of my own pocket, on this occasion it was the Communist Party that had to fork out for our accommodation. This political body saves where it can, and apparently had done so on the eighteen doctors it had requested to come over in order to study Chen-chiu – acupuncture in western terminology.

It is remarkable that even the Chinese talk to us of 'acupuncture' for the most part, although they should know better. However, few of them really understand foreign languages, including all sorts of western languages, and they simply copy what is found in dictionaries – which very often is not correct. For this reason, they translate the two characters 'Chen' 針 (needle application) and 'Chiu' 灸 (herbal moxibustion) without any differentiation, and incorrectly, simply as 'acupuncture'. But no one else has noticed the irregularity so far.

Dr Haubensack and I occupied a double room. After dinner, we talked about what we intended to do on our evenings in Shanghai. He thought about something exotic – for instance, about amusing himself with a pretty Chinese girl, he and she going out together and ending up in a gloomy bar and dancing to romantic music. Taken up with this for a moment, he hummed a melody to himself softly – 'Nu de Chine, nu caline, nu d'amour...' It was something from the operetta *The Land of Smiles* (German: *Das Land des Lächelns*). He didn't know yet that here there was no such music and there were certainly no bars. Modern China's taste in these matters is quite different from that of the West. It does not share nineteenth- and early-twentieth-century European tastes. The music that blares from a thousand amplifiers all over the place in this city is shrill and in no way sweet or romantic, but primitive and even aggressive. Apparently, it is what is regarded as 'revolutionary', since it moves to the rhythms of the march, proceeding ever forward towards its object, undeterred, like Mao Tse-tung's soldiers on the Long March to eventual conquest.

At that very moment I heard my neighbour cursing in the shower, telling me that the tap didn't work. When it was turned on, an ice-cold stream of water shot straight into the user's face and over his clothes. There was no warm water. Exactly the same happened to me three years ago. Clearly, it was intended to mean: 'Welcome to you, western guest! Welcome, you decadent capitalist, to our enormously more advanced Chinese People's Republic!'

We recalled that we had been dumped here in this double room against our express wishes and, in passing, had been promised that we would receive separate apartments in Shanghai. This, we had replied, was the least that could be offered to two established medical specialists who, furthermore, were the delegates of their respective governments and were thus acting in what one might call a semi-diplomatic capacity, representing two different states.

As if pulled out of water, Haubensack appeared from the bathroom.

'Merde! If things go on like this, I'll be catching the next plane home!' He had placed a photo of his pretty wife on the bedside table immediately on arrival and was already badly missing home.

Speaking from experience, I prophesied that it would continue to go on like this. 'Small repair jobs in hotels not usually are attended to, and in other matters, as well, negligence and mess is the order of the day. In this, the Chinese are quite generous,' I added.

'Generous? Ugh!' he snarled. 'Damned shambles! That's what it is! And I can't even change, because my bags that I checked in at Geneva still haven't arrived. What kind of damn place is this?'

I had lent him some of my underwear, and because his luggage had not yet arrived, he had been wearing the same bespoke Paris suit that he had worn on boarding the plane in Geneva. After twenty hours in the aircraft, it was badly creased and urgently needed ironing.

'It's at least a good omen, my friend, that on arrival you were "baptised" with relatively clean Chinese water,' I said, by way of calming him down. 'On the very first day of my medical career I was similarly soused with something very different!'

'With what, then?'

'At the beginning of my practical training I had to get up at five in the morning and be ready for duty at six at the hospital, which was under the auspices of the Free University of Berlin. I was allotted to a group of nurses and sisters, and my first job was to fetch the urine flasks from the men's ward which had been filled overnight. These so-called ducks I had to take to a certain toilette, empty them and clean them. How was this done? A young apprentice nurse showed me with the flask she had in her hand.

' "You've gotta do it this way," she said while I watched her carefully. "An' then push the thing up with force exactly under the swill-tap nozzle."

'I did what she showed me. But the little bitch had put the thing in the wrong way round in order to make a fool of me. The powerful stream of water swished into the air, made a large arc, and the contents of the whole bottle doused me from head to foot. Everyone cheered.

' "Great!" the small crowd around me roared in unison. "Now 'e's baptised with piss, and what better for a good doctor?"

'This "baptism" went round the hospital like a house on fire and I became well known overnight, as it were. Apart from that, as one baptised in urine, I enjoyed certain privileges such as, for example, extra rations nicked by nurses from the kitchen, and at the end of the training I received a particularly good mark for my labours and the added note that I was very well suited for my profession, and all this because of the above-mentioned incident.'

Dr Haubensack grinned and composed himself a little.

Beer from Qingdao

I suggested we go down to the restaurant to drink something. Still pretty wet from his unbidden baptism, and still grumbling under his breath, he followed me outside. Once in the corridor we had to wait almost fifteen minutes for the lift to finally arrive. It had trundled past our level on a number of occasions, however, and it was clear that someone apparently possessed a special lift key with which he or she could guide the lift to stop at a desired storey and so prevent it stopping at intermediate floors on the way. Later, we learned that this was nothing unusual, and that high-ranking party officials were at liberty to use the lift in this way in China's hotels. In comparison, then, were we mere second-class people or folks of inferior quality – or perhaps even a kind of bourgeois pest in the eyes of the communist big shots?

The restaurant was dimly lit and smelled thickly of cooking fat. I was used to it. For me, it was what I had come to call the 'Chinese Stink'. Every country, I had discovered, had its own particular odour. If one were to cover my eyes and place me in India, for example, I could tell you whether I was in

Madras, Delhi, Bombay or Calcutta. The same would be true of the Paris Métro, London's Underground, Hong Kong, Mexico City or Amsterdam – even Copenhagen or Stockholm. Every place exuded its own specific, characteristic smell. Incidentally, every human being has his or her own olfactory attributes too. During my professional career, this olfactory sensitivity of mine had often helped me in discerning certain diseases.

We sat down. We were the only guests. Behind the bar two waiters in dirty yellow jackets were talking to each other. One of them had stretched his arms over the counter and was swaying backwards and forwards on his stool. Neither disguised his utter contempt for westerners. We waited.

'This is going on forever,' said my companion in some annoyance. 'How do you call the waiter in Chinese?'

I delved into the recesses of my mind. After all, it had been over three years since I was in the country.

'Wei Tong-zhi,' I called. 'Comrade, come over here.'

One of them looked over to us, pulled back his arms from the counter in slow motion, sat upright, held up his head, cleared his throat loudly, collected sufficient slime in his mouth to spit it into what looked very much like an enamel chamber pot under the stool, looked long at what had been discharged, and then strolled over comfortably to our table.

'Nimen hao,' he said.

'What did he say?' Haubensack asked.

'He wished us a good evening,' I replied.

'He'd do better to bring us two beers.'

'Lai liang bei pi-ju', I said, translating for my companion.

After I had spoken to the waiter in Chinese, he reacted a trifle quicker than before and went away. Another ten minutes passed. Then he returned with a large bottle of Qingdao beer and two glasses, threw a rusty bottle-opener noisily on the table and removed himself without another word.

'Does that mean that we have to open the bottle ourselves?' my colleague asked.

'Well, I imagine so. Here, in the paradise for soldiers, farmers and workers, it's pretty much the rule.'

'Well damn me!' Haubensack cursed. 'Some rotten paradise!'

The beer was lukewarm. There was not the slightest foam on it. But it was delicious.

'Actually, it's German beer,' I ventured. 'Qingdao was a German colony before the First World War. Many Germans lived there, and one of their number was the priest Richard Wilhelm who produced the best translations from Chinese, better than all the western sinologists put together: Lao-Tse's

Dao-De-Jing, the *Spring and Autumn Annals* of Confucius, the *Book of Changes* (the *Yi-Jing*), and a whole lot more. But by far the most important thing to happen was that German masters of the art of brewing beer came over to the town and from then on brewed a beer which is still drinkable.'

'And we're expected to drink this warm stuff?' Haubensack grumbled. 'I much prefer my Strasbourg Mutzig.'

'In an emergency, it is said, the Devil will eat flies. At least the stuff's fluid.'

'Really?' Haubensack countered. 'So we'll get flies for our next meal?'

'Could well be. According to an old Chinese saying, "Every creature that presents its back to the sun is edible."'

'That's applicable to flies.'

'Yes,' I agreed. 'Human beings are excepted though, but if they did in fact put their backs to the sun, their flesh would end up in a soup or be served as a rissole. Cheers, my friend!'

We sucked at our beer and thought of Europe.

'Into what kind of hole have we fallen, I'd like to know?' Haubensack said irritably. 'I can smell it; something's not quite right in this country. It's somehow uncanny. I've been around quite a bit, but here there are still a lot of nasty surprises in store for us.'

'Well, I wouldn't say that. We'll get used to it. And we want to learn about Chen-chiu.'

Mao and European Acupuncture

'Why do you always say "Chen-chiu" and not acupuncture?' my colleague asked me.

'Because that's the correct term for what we're about to learn. The Chinese have called it "Chen-chiu" for several thousand years. "Acupuncture" is a European concept and therefore a European invention.'

'But they talk to us about acupuncture. Why do they do that?'

'Because they don't know any other language than Chinese. Few Chinese ever really master English, French, German or Spanish. They cannot spell words written in letters of our alphabet and cannot understand the linguistic roots of our languages since our alphabet and its letters are something entirely alien to them. They only know characters. They merely take the western translations of their own characters from a dictionary as gospel, however false this translation might be. It's quite impossible to "spell" Chinese. Chinese is a picture language. I think I've already mentioned this. I once had a Chinese medical employee, a doctor with a university degree from Shanghai. He frightened all my female patients who had reached their climacteric by describing them as having now reached their "crematorium". In pronunciation, the most difficult thing for them all is to differentiate an "l" from an "r". Most of them never learn it.'

In this connection, there is the story of the English journalist on a visit to Mao Tse-tung, whom he regarded as a democratic politician, and whom he asked , 'When did you have your last election?'

Typically, Mao, like all Chinese, confused the pronunciation of 'l' and 'r' and said, 'This morning.'

Haubensack took a long swig at his warm beer. 'Oh, Lord,' he sighed. 'Things can only get worse!'

'Well, perhaps,' I went on, 'the majority of Chinese can no longer read their own ancient pictographs stemming from the old form of writing. About twenty years ago, Mao Tse-tung had reduced many of the characters to simpler forms so that those under fifty-five, say, can no longer read the old forms and so can't understand what they mean. This is also true for the younger Chinese doctors, and they find themselves tapping around in the dark as far as this is concerned.'

'And why did Mr Mao do that?'

'He probably did it because he wanted to stamp out the connections between today's Chinese and the roots of their culture. In ancient times China had the most beautiful culture in the world. But Mao himself wanted to be the only Chinese god, although there were never gods in historic China in the western sense of that word.'

'Incredible!'

'It was for this reason that a western doctor – a psychiatrist travelling in China about ten years ago and writing about Chinese medicine – had to find something god-like comparable to Mao Tse-tung in human history. He went back to the origin of religions – to the prophets and lawgivers of ancient times – to make such a comparison. For example, this man cited Moses and the Promised Land, Jesus Christ, the Son of God, or the conquest of half the world under the banner of Mohammed to support his absurd thesis that these historical events had been excelled by those having recently taken place in mainland China, in the lifetime of a single individual – Mao Tse-tung.'

'This flatly contradicts the processes of Enlightenment in Europe. Are the Chinese really so stupid nowadays?'

'Political contradiction here leads to imprisonment, torture or even execution.'

'This kind of nonsense is a typical psychiatrist's attitude. We know the type

– not the slightest knowledge of medicine but a big mouth with not much substance.'

'I do know one or two sensible people in this field, but these are rare, and you're right. Actually, I had opportunity to work in that area and was an assistant once in a psychiatric ward.'

'I don't know any sensible ones.'

'Today, there are many comparisons between Mao and the great founders of religions. An American pastor and religious scientist has even gone so far as to assert that religions in China, even those which were suspended in the past, have coalesced today into new forms of religious feeling among the Chinese. He maintains that the commands of the Maoist regime have taken on a sacred character. The demands to cooperate with the regime's objectives have an almost religious significance – for example, the Marxist-Leninist books distributed by this "Chairman" have, he says, the distinction of holy texts in which a pious people can find the answer to every question which might trouble them.'

'Mass conditioning kept in motion by violence and political organisation … ?'

'This seems to be rather a kind of brainwashing.'

'We'll see.'

'This psychiatrist went on to say that in modern China Mao is honoured and respected without requiring churches and altars. There is no need to attribute divine qualities to him, since he embodies the characteristics of politicians such as the Americans Thomas Jefferson, George Washington and Abraham Lincoln, or men like Ralph Waldo Emerson, all in one. So it's not unusual to come across simple people in China who revere Mao as a kind of god.'

'Sickening.' Haubensack shook himself. 'I've never come across such books.'

'Essentially, Mao, as the result of western communist influence, especially that of Stalin's Soviet communism, was something of a perverted character, a Chinese who deliberately cheated on his own culture.'

Haubensack took another long quaff at his warm beer. 'Mao as someone perverted by the West; I've never heard that before!'

'You won't find it in western newspapers.'

'I know too little about modern Chinese politics, but I simply refer to the ancient history and to a few recent books.'

'The old history of China was very different.'

'It would have been better for Mao to have introduced our western alphabet into the country. This awful way of writing is perhaps the actual curtain behind which the Chinese have lain hidden for so long.'

'Well, but we have also to recognise that this way of writing was the cultural, and above all the political, instrument with which the "Middle Kingdom" – in other words, the Han culture and its surrounding satellite states – could be ruled at all, and that for thousands of years. This vehicle of communication was that which took China's cultural achievements as far as Korea and from there to Japan and even as far as Europe. After all, much has been translated and handed down to us.'

'Was changing the traditional Chinese characters a demagogic trick, then?' asked Haubensack. 'Or why did he do that?'

'Mao wanted to destroy the link that existed between the younger generation and the old Chinese culture. One called this in its broadest application a "Cultural Revolution". We're still in the middle of it. I experienced this in 1965 in Canton, and then later indirectly in Cambodia and Vietnam. At that time I worked in Hong Kong and used to travel around South East Asia in my free time. On my last trip to China three years ago, I heard that the Cultural Revolution was still abroad and as vital as ever, but today it is called the "Gang of Four". We will probably hear more of this later.'

'Can you give me an example of the influence the shortened form of Chinese writing had on people and politics?'

'Let's take a general example which is well known everywhere – the pictogram for "love", 愛 Ai. Mao removed the element "heart", 心 Xin, from the pictograph. Today, the character "love" in Chinese is only 爱, and this has a significant impact for the people in mainland China.'

'Does that mean that "love" in China nowadays is without heart?'

'For the Communist Party the human heart is an unpredictable factor. Love is something which is only felt for its "Great Chairman" and the party itself. Deep feelings of love between a man and a woman are politically not desirable, because the result of such situation could be too many children. The party strictly presides over the one-child marriage.'

'I've heard about that,' Haubensack nodded. 'But why didn't the West understand China and the whole of the Far East? Does what you say go for Chinese medicine as well? Give me an example.'

'I've already given you one: acupuncture. It's a wrong term because the second element of Chen-chiu, warming with moxa, just isn't there. Europeans only think of needle treatment when they hear or read the word acupuncture. The Chinese, however, understand a treatment as having a number of facets in its application, implying various techniques and methods of treatment. There are other irregularities, too. Take the so-called meridians as referred to in western rendering. The word "meridian" represents an idea taken from geography. But in western acupuncture it is used to denote the blood vessels and nerve pathways in the human organism – in other words, it is used for structures we get to know in our first term at medical college. These "Jing-mai" or "Jing-luo" are nothing more than the pulsating vessels of the human organism. Only in this way can the Chinese pulse diagnosis be logically explained: by the evaluation of the pulsating arteries, thus making medical sense. Our well-known nerves and arteries are actually the transfer paths of acupuncture effects. The meridians of geography, on the other hand, the lines of longitude on the globe, have nothing to do with blood pulsation and acupuncture at all. Try to "diagnose" a line passing through Greenwich with your palpating fingers – that's pure idiocy. Neither I nor the whole congregation of Chinese doctors past and present could do such a thing!'

'I can see that of course,' my companion replied. 'But do you really mean that we in the West have never really understood China?'

'Let's look at German doctors, as an example. A little while ago, I informed the medical representative for my area that, under the auspices of the German Ministry for Health, I would be going to Shanghai for four months to study acupuncture and so would have to ask for temporary suspension from emergency duty. This request was summarily dismissed. I had been told that as a registered doctor in my city I had always to be on call during my duty days and nights. Accordingly, there was no question of my staying for any length of time in China.

'The president of our local board of representatives, a man with a pig face, whom I had personally elected and to whom I therefore had faithfully turned for assistance, asked me:

"Where do you want to go, to China? These folks still wear plaits, don't they? What the devil do you want to do there? It's an underdeveloped country!"

"I want to study acupuncture there."

"You'd do better to go to the United States or to Sweden. There, they have an advanced medicine. In China you'll find nothing to your advantage."

"The German government has commissioned me to study acupuncture in China and so provided for me to stay in that country."

"We have nothing to do with this government."

In order to emphasise his importance, he puffed out his massive thorax, which showed suspicious signs of wind in the lungs, emphysema.

"We're a public medical corporation, you know," he hissed, "and as such we have our own jurisdiction, the local medical court of law."

'This latter above all seemed to lend certainty to his statement.

'He looked at me in a way which threatened to apprehend me immediately and drag me before the medical court to be condemned as a deserter of my duties.

'"I am adhering to the rules of the medical profession," I said.

'"I'm not so sure of that," the fat one retorted. "Acupuncture is not an acknowledged area of medical activity, and health insurance policies don't pay a penny for it. You, on the other hand, carry it out in your practice and I regard this with a jaundiced eye."

'"What am I suspected of, then?"

'"Of odd convictions and a not particularly stable psychological condition. You understand, I hope, what I mean?"

'"The health insurance companies will eventually have to change their opinion."

'"So – you think so. Under the word 'acupuncture' in my dictionary one can read a most plausible explanation – namely, that it is 'The piecemeal breaking up of the foetus during a complicated birth.' For that you don't need to go to China. You can learn this here in Germany."

'"Your dictionary is out of date."

'He gave me a poisonous look. "You'll carry out your emergency duties here on the dot. We're not going to give you leave of absence."

'Officially, there the matter rested. I went to China despite him, since I was convinced that I was on the track of something absolutely new in medicine.'

Our beer was coming to an end and we didn't really want to go for another bottle. So we took the lift to our room, where we discovered that Haubensack's luggage, after two days' delay, had at last arrived.

Our second night in the Middle Kingdom would, we hoped, be a restful one, but this was not to be so. The glaring lights of traffic lit up our room. The noise from the busy street below, the hooting and the stream of cars and other vehicles grinding by, kept us awake. Other unpleasant things also disturbed us. I awoke and made out a dark figure slipping from one point to another in the room. Nobody had knocked. This shadow flitted to the cupboard, opened it noisily, looked inside, rummaged through the things in it and then slipped away again as quietly as it had come. I tried to flick on the light, but no light came, then I got out of bed and went to the door to lock it, but there was no key. I wanted to look in the cupboard, but that had been locked. However, from inside I could hear a kind of clucking sound coming from a machine of some sort. 'Are we being bugged?' I asked myself.

Our Medical Group

In the course of the last few days we have all made each other's acquaintance. There are two doctors from Switzerland who generally speak French with one another, but who speak German to me. Then there are the two colleagues from Holland, Adrienne Coningk and Alice Van Anholt, who are both women doctors, one specialising in anaesthesia, the other in paediatrics, who speak to one another in Dutch, but to me in French or in German. Then there is Dr Haubensack, a colleague from Lorraine in France, who speaks to me in German and to the others in French, and when he comes across Alsatians, he speaks to them in his home dialect, as he did this morning in the foyer of the hotel after breakfast. Another anaesthetist and consultant at a clinic in Paris called the Hopital Necker is there. His name is Dr Lagarde.

Two colleagues from Laos have beardless children's faces and it is difficult to assess how old they are. Both speak French, but use their native language to converse with each other. Then there are two dark-skinned doctors from Cameroon, one of whom runs around in an old, greasy khaki uniform which is too tight for him. He looks more like an army officer, a military doctor with the rank of captain perhaps. He grins and laughs whenever he can. Apparently he's an 'odd bod', as the English say, a joker ever ready for a lark, whose name is Adnan Kirinin. The other, whose name is Balu, wears a colourful toga which reaches to the ground and his head is turbanned with a similar many-coloured, round headdress, which I can make out neither as a hat nor a cap. He's ready to tell everyone he is the son of an African chieftain and thereby allows himself airs and graces.

The two from Cameroon talk to each other in their native language, at other times in stumbling French, and they can also speak some English. Apart from these, there are two very tall Africans from Chad. These two are introverted and quiet. One never sees them laugh and they seldom take part in general conversation.

Three other colleagues are from Syria. One of these is the consultant in charge of an anaesthesia department in Damascus who has already informed me that for some time now he has been applying acupuncture techniques and once attended a fourteen-day introductory course in applying needle anaesthesia in operations. This was undertaken in the People's Republic. All of them speak to us in French, but converse in Arabic among themselves.

The three Syrians and the two Africans from Chad all eat at the same, specially prepared table because they are Muslims and don't eat pork. The Syrian anaesthetist, the corpulent military doctor and I are the only ones in the group of eighteen who have been to China before. For this reason we are referred to by the staff as 'Lao Pengyou' – 'old friends'.

There is an Ethiopian nurse in the group who cannot participate in our general studies from tomorrow onwards because she cannot speak French, only a little English. Added to this, she doesn't possess comparable qualifications and so will be allotted to a group of people studying acupuncture who are not medically qualified. Apparently, non-medically qualified people – that is to say, paramedics and medical personnel and even laymen – are entitled to be instructed in acupuncture and moxibustion therapy in today's China. This has certain advantages for the Chinese. Both professional groups are strictly separated from one another. We were to learn why later.

Here, we can speak of a 'pigeon-hole' bureaucracy where everything runs according to forms and norms that have been previously planned and regulated, but which for us are not at all transparent, since no one on the Chinese side discloses the slightest detail about what is going on. Everything requires a 'paper', whether it be for the purchase of a particular piece of material, an excursion into the neighbourhood or a personal encounter with a Chinese colleague if these lie outside the planned order of procedure. These 'papers' are signed by the party superior and stamped as official permission which one must submit on going through the many controls, presided over by green-uniformed soldiers or by men who belong to a special cadre of official personnel dressed in black Mao tunics and trousers.

Today, the third day of our stay, we were in the so-called Forbidden City in which can be seen the Imperial Palace, which I visited three years ago while following the usual tourists' programme. No one can get to know China in this way, however. Nevertheless, the majority of tourists go through this controlled procedure and are apparently content with such demonstrations. For their part, the Chinese can control groups of people better than they can control individuals. Control! This is their magic word and one of the main activities of the party. I was particularly interested in that room of the palace where the emperor, Huang-Di, is said to have interviewed ongoing Chen-chiu physicians and enjoined them long ago to keep their oath of professional good conduct. I took the opportunity of asking Dr Cai about this on our circuit through the palace. Dr Cai is a high-ranking doctor in the service of the Ministry of Health. This man's face was a faded yellow, and his cheeks pockmarked. He was tall, stiff and pale, a man of few words, but when he spoke he did so in explosive gusts through the nose, an altogether unhealthy appearance. He knew nothing of the historical text and nothing even of the book *Ling-Shu-Jing.* He knew nothing either about the doctor's oath in ancient China and did not have anything to say about the room used for such purposes. But he did say that Beijing at this time when these scripts were set down was not yet the capital of China. It could well have been, therefore, that the writings had their origin in Huang Di's palace situated somewhere else and possibly in another town altogether. This Dr Cai, who spoke good French, was to escort us in a plane to Shanghai the day after tomorrow and there direct us to the College of Chinese Medicine.

On our return to the hotel, I bumped into my former interpreter on the steps who had assisted me three years before, a certain Mr Zhu. I had found him a helpful and well-informed individual who had looked after me during my visit and who had also given me a Chinese name, La Lo-be – a name I had since then printed on my Chinese visiting cards. At first, he didn't seem to recognise me or did not want to recognise me. I had no 'paper' with me that would have facilitated a conversation with him. The danger of being constantly controlled, something which affects not only foreign visitors, but also Chinese people themselves should they not be high-ranking party members, clearly embarrassed him. For this reason, he felt it better to feign ignorance of our acquaintance. His attitude was most odd, especially in view of the fact that only years ago we had spent almost four weeks in each other's company, had travelled together through China and had had a good deal of fun doing so. He had always called me 'Doctor, Doctor' and, moreover, constantly repeated that I was the very first western doctor whom he had had the pleasure of accompanying on a journey through the country. Perhaps he couldn't place me at first considering he had had so many people to look after on visits to China. However, when he realised who I was, he was clearly on edge. He pressed me into a shadowed corner of the staircase where no one could see us, put out his fingers to briefly shake hands and then whispered, 'Doctor, Doctor…', laughing nervously and showing the whites of his teeth. It seemed that he wanted to wish me well, because he kept saying, 'All the best, all the best…' Then, as suddenly as he had appeared, he was off again as if swallowed up by the earth itself. I would have been so glad to have exchanged a few words with him. The fact was that he would not have been allowed to enter into conversation with me. And as for me, I was later to learn why all this was so and, furthermore, why the average communist was obliged to keep to the rules.

Varying Opinions about Acupuncture (Chen-chiu)

It was our third day in Beijing, and after breakfast we got to know each other a little better. We asked what it was that was so special about Chinese 'acupuncture' and the so-called needle anaesthesia derived from it that had recently aroused so much interest in the West, making it something of a sensation. We were alone – or so we thought. Somewhere, however, there were hidden microphones, that was for sure, and we were being recorded. The interpreters' collective would evaluate the conversations later on.

'Well, my friends, I ask you: is there anything in this business? Or is the whole thing a political bluff? Perhaps it's nothing more than suggestion or the placebo effect? We know at least that such things are real enough.'

This is what did the rounds at this moment as we sat there asking each other the same questions. We were all thinking about needle anaesthetic techniques in apparent use during operations. This is what we were here to learn about so that we could use it in our clinics at home.

One of our two colleagues from the Netherlands, the blonde, Adrienne Coningk from Leiden, had already gained some knowledge of these techniques. She had been a student at the Association Française d'Acupuncture in Paris, where she had worked together with others on such projects. 'If you ask me,' she said, 'the whole thing is a load of Chinese claptrap. In Paris, they talk about some kind of imaginary energy that runs along meridians of some kind – that's to say, along channels in the human body as yet undiscovered by western medicine. There's no such thing. If there was, how come we have studied modern medicine for so long and been able to help thousands of patients? If that's what they want to do with us here, then we're off back to Holland at the next opportunity, Alice and I. As doctors we have enough to do and at home we're needed every hour. In other words, we can't just mark time here. So, if we have nothing sensible and practical to learn, you won't be seeing me and Alice Van Anholt for much longer.'

Someone in our midst said, 'On the other hand, perhaps we could all find a new usable theory for this form of medicine.'

At that point, Haubensack cut in, 'Listen, friends, I've been operating for the last twenty years every day and have been faced with every kind of surgical situation you can think of. As a result I'm familiar with the human body as a whole and my scalpel has investigated every corner of the human organism. When necessary, I do transplantations as well. If there were such "meridians" or "channels" like those suggested here, I would have certainly come across them. In my transplanted kidneys, for example, there's certainly nothing of the kind to be found. Or what do you think? This stuff about meridians is pure crap. I've been talking to Ralf Rompard about all this.'

Then Adnan Kirinin, the African from Cameroon in the khaki uniform, spoke up. He went on to explain in halting French that 'we shouldn't forget that our modern medicine is far from understanding everything there is to know about things medical and human health. I practise medicine in darkest Africa and often enough my work takes me far inland in the course of looking after pygmies there. These people are small and their heads barely reach to my navel. But medically they are geniuses. They know of herbal recipes, which, often enough, have remarkable effects. But they don't want to tell me about them. On the other hand, Mao Tse-tung has managed to bring Chinese doctors to reveal their traditional secrets for the benefit of humanity. I'm sure we can learn something from our stay here.'

This Dr Kirinin had already spent a year here in Beijing learning about Chinese medicine and for this reason was well disposed to China. At the time of speaking he was one of the directors of the regional hospital in Yaunde. His French was poor and difficult for us to understand. Nevertheless, he gave one the impression of being absolutely honest, and was convinced of what he says. In addition, he seemed to be very intelligent.

'Think about it for a moment, friends.' It was the voice of one of the Swiss in our company, a surgical consultant from a hospital in Lausanne. 'Are we to give up a form of medicine which has changed the world for a primitive half-digested ancient theory?'

Everyone was in agreement with this: No!

'Well, wait a bit, my countryman,' said his Swiss colleague. 'Could it be that we're totally blinded by our daily "successes" in practice – especially you surgeons? You operate here and there and then the patient is apparently cured of his ailment. The fact is that we just cannot imagine anything else than our established form of medicine and for this reason are not in a position to offer anything not falling within that constellation of thought. Here, we have a chance to add a new dimension to medicine in the West. It's lying in front of us and we have the good fortune to be the first in line to receive it.'

The Syrian doctor chipped in at this point to comment, 'Well, as a practising anaesthetist I have to say from experience that the implementation of pain-reducing acupuncture functions perfectly well. I use this in operating, too, though less frequently these days. However, I have to tell you that I've been using this technique of pain-reducing needle therapy for three years now.'

'Is that a real anaesthesia in the classical medical sense?' Haubensack asked.

The woman doctor from the Netherlands was equally doubtful. 'I can't really imagine this to be the case. While on the operating table, patients wouldn't keep still. They would move about and twitch with pain. I wouldn't trust myself to anaesthetise patients in this way for my surgeons. At best, one creates a hypalgesia – in other words, a reduced sensitivity to pain. A trace of the pain will always still be there, so to speak. Patients would have to feel something!'

'In Germany, our colleague Rompard has been using acupuncture for some years,' Haubensack intervened.

I then told those assembled about my own experiences over the last five years in my practice. I told them that I had treated migraine and backache, cured asthma, and even managed to break down kidney stones, cured sleeplessness and been able to restore mental balance in my patients.

'If that functions as you say, then we ought to find a scientific explanation for it,' said Adrienne.

'We want to do just that!' In this everyone agreed.

My colleagues were now interested in what I had to offer as far as acupuncture theories were concerned.

'Do you mean the so-called points in acupuncture and moxa therapy don't exist either?' Haubensack, with whom I had already discussed the problem before, asked me.

'Quite so. The "Xue-Wei", the original Chinese term for it, means the tiny canals connecting one part of human organism with another by leading into the deepest parts of the body's interior. The depth of this "interior" of the human organism was something quite well known to ancient Chinese doctors. According to an old text – namely, the book *Su-Wen* – they were referred to as the 365 "Luo" – that is, the 365 small vessels making up a network. For us, they are the blood vessels and nerve paths. After all, we have to acknowledge that the Chinese doctors were the first in medical history to practise anatomy from a scientific point of view and to dissect and research the human body and, as far as they were able, to remarkably illustrate their findings.'

'Why 365?' asked Dr. Sifferlin, the Swiss surgeon.

'That is the number of days in a year. Ancient Chinese medicine tried to create understanding for the cosmic order of the universe, for the world and for man. For them at the time, this was the encompassing order to be found in nature.'

'How do you know all this?' the French Claude Giroudoux wondered.

'Because I have for some time been studying classical Chinese texts and analysing ancient Chinese characters.'

'If that's the case, why have you come to China once again?' Adrienne Coningk wanted to know.

'In order to get to know the current situation better. I want to be able to understand the present political situation and be able, too, to come into direct conversation with Chinese people. Apart from this, I want to find out whether in some corner of modern China there is something of the ancient traditional medical culture still alive.'

'You're quite clearly an optimist!' It sounded almost like an accusation.

The majority of participants, although doctors of long professional standing, were mere beginners as far as acupuncture was concerned, Achille Haubensack included. Back in our hotel room he took up his theme again with enthusiasm.

'When I get back to Nancy and Metz with my diploma, I can hang it on my door: "Qualified Acupuncturist, Shanghai". After which, patients will just storm the doors ... There's no one I know in Lorraine who can sport knowledge of this therapy.'

We had learned that we would have to go through an official examination after four months and, if we passed, we would receive an official certificate from the People's Republic of China qualifying us to practise acupuncture worldwide. I prophesied that Haubensack would give up his surgical practice and only practise acupuncture, because it was so fascinating. But he would hear none of it.

'I'm a good surgeon,' he told me, 'that's enough. I've learned to operate well, having studied the business thoroughly in Strasbourg, Paris and Basel. If you ever come to visit me in Nancy, you are cordially invited to watch me operate and look on as long as you please. You can even assist me if you wish. After all, you've learned something of the art yourself, have you not?' As an Alsatian he pronounced the word 'Nancy' not as a Frenchman would, but as 'Nansish'. On the other hand, I admired his French. He spoke it as perfectly as he spoke German, and apart from these languages he could also speak English and Spanish, and was familiar with ancient Greek and Latin from his school days.

The next day I would have to give a welcoming speech in French, and consequently I had to prepare the whole thing minutely, typing the manuscript and having it ready to read off, all of which comprised a special job for me over the next few hours. I had asked to address the audience in English, but this request had been dismissed with the objection that French had been the official language agreed upon in setting up the course. In these matters, too, the Chinese are very finicky. The plan has to be kept to, even to the smallest detail.

At the Embassy

That afternoon I was at the German embassy, that for West Germany, the Chinese dealing with our course emphasised. In these concerns, too, they were extremely accurate, and in my opinion overcorrect. In other words, I was not in China as a German, but only as a West German. There was a second Germany, the so-called German Democratic Republic, which is ruled by a communist government and therefore to be preferred by the Mainland Chinese.

I had got to know the woman who was the diplomat for cultural matters at Beijing Airport, where she had greeted me as the representative of the German Ministry of Health. She now introduced me to the ambassador. This gentleman was known not only as a diplomat, but also as a writer. He was in his early sixties, and had a good knowledge of China which went back to the '30s. He looked grey, everything on him was grey: his face, his hair, his suit, his tie, even his pale lips which he constantly pressed tightly together and against each other in a quite sour way. When he smiled, which was rarely, his face assumed a grotesque grimace. His manner was very matter-of-fact, but at the same time he showed personal interest in many things, above all in Chinese medicine. I told him why I had come over to China to study in Shanghai. He listened for a long time …

'It's probable that things won't turn out in the way you expect,' he said. 'For this reason I'll give you a piece of advice. If something doesn't comply with your wishes in Shanghai, write to me and tell me all about the problem in full detail. Register the letter. Long before the letter reaches me here in Beijing, the problem, whatever it is, will have been solved and the business regulated to your satisfaction. The reason for this is that here in China nobody wants to lose face under any circumstances.'

I was astonished at this. Apparently, he knew his Chinese very well: 'Each letter you mail in China is read by the security officials and reacted to immediately.' I then asked him whether I could ring him from Shanghai should I have any reason to do so. With a wink, he said it was theoretically possible. 'This has almost the same effect as a letter,' he said, 'so think carefully about what you want to say on the phone. Every telephone conversation is tapped, every letter is opened, and it's probable that your rooms are all wired up. But anyway, you can adjust yourself to that.'

How, exactly?

'You'll find that out yourself in time,' he said.

Outside, the lady diplomat received me with the words, 'You were a long time in there. Usually he's short and to the point with people.'

'He wanted to hear something about Chinese medicine.'

She spoke a little more softly than the ambassador. 'Diplomatic staff here are pretty lonely. We live, if you like, in a kind of ghetto. We are only allowed to mix among our own kind. Apart from necessary contacts, we have no intercourse at all with the Chinese. For this reason, I have a lot of time on my hands. I have read almost all Mao Tse-tung's works. His books, you see, have been translated into practically every language. It's not great literature and certainly not a philosophy, and everything anyway is second hand. Much of it stems from the old Chinese ways of thinking, and all this is arbitrarily mixed together with Marx, Engels and Lenin, often enough in a pretty artless way. These days I've left that stuff to read Lao Tse, Confucius and Chuang-tse. I even try to understand them in the original, but it is difficult. In the evening I sit and paint Chinese characters. This seems to help me even physically. I can feel the power inherent in these characters.'

'What do you think of Chinese medicine?'

'You understand more about this as a specialist in the field.'

'Have you ever been treated by a Chinese doctor?'

'Yes, and it did me good. On the other hand, I hate this impersonal anonymity in Chinese clinics. I can't think that this is in line with what the old masters of Chinese healing felt and practised.'

'I agree with you.'

'Here, one is just a number in the mass at large. Even as a qualified foreign diplomat from a "friendly country", as the phrase has it – in other words, as a representative of another state. Everyone here serves the masses, the people – but not the individual.'

'In ancient times it was different. In the book *Ling-Shu-Jing*, for example, we read quite the opposite: "Of all that lives between Heaven and Earth, human life is the most important."'

'I don't know that particular work, but it would seem to be the kind of general wisdom of this wonderful country.'

In the visitors' room of the embassy there was suddenly a certain atmosphere that captured the flow of time, the inner life of the world, so to speak. Was it possible that this German diplomat, who was so interested in Chinese tradition, actually understood more about ancient Chinese culture than the Chinese themselves today?

I, too, will get hold of a brush, paper and ink and produce Chinese characters when I stay in Shanghai.

At the conclusion of our chat, I mentioned an unpleasant experience I had had at a Beijing bank. In compliance with the German Foreign Office and the Ministry of Health, I had bought a number of travellers' cheques in US dollars, so as to be able to change them into China's currency.

However, when I got to the bank I was told that American travellers' cheques were no longer acceptable. Why?

The reason for this, she informed me, was that America was trading with Taiwan and this was a kind of act of revenge on the part of communist China for these transactions. China is able to do this through its banks as it is not bound by contractual law to comply with the terms of international money transfer and currency exchange.

For me personally, it was not a large sum, but as a customer one looks a fool in these circumstances. In essence, it is a political move which makes use of artificial, managed unpleasantness such as this in order to make foreign guests aware of what is going on in the broader political field. I sat there like an idiot with my cheques and felt indignant that I could not move because of some incident abroad involving the Americans and the Chinese. I thought about the matter for a moment. I realised as I did so that this was exactly what the Chinese authorities wanted to achieve. We have to understand their socialism. We have to think in terms of economic developments, but do they think so far themselves?

'Were you ever in Taiwan yourself?' the diplomat asked me.

'Yes, at the end of the '60s.'

'Did you like it there?'

'Very much.'

'Don't tell anybody here about that,' she said.

'I have a second passport with a Taiwan and a US visa.'

'Well, I hope you haven't got them with you here', she went on. 'You could find yourself in big trouble. So please be careful. Mao's republic will certainly change in future, but for the moment it's still a place full of surprises!'

The Great Wall and a Dead Dog

On the fourth day we were transported in an ancient, swinging bus over dusty, rough country roads to the imperial graves of the Ming era and to the Great Wall in the north. This was a tourist route on which I'd travelled before. As soon as we had left Beijing's city boundaries, the driver of this jalopy gradually increased speed and began to sing revolutionary songs with gusto. The suspension of this ancient thing was practically non-existent and we were thrown violently from side to side and up and down until our bones ached. Suddenly, the man at the wheel braked hard, and the brakes protested. A dull thud. The bus stopped. What had happened? The driver and

Dr Cai, who was sitting next to him at the front, got out together. The driver, a pale-faced young fellow in uniform and with the high cheekbones of a Mongol, went round the bus excitedly, lay down in the dust, pushed himself under the bus and returned with a black bundle: a dead dog. He had been driving too fast and run it over, poor thing.

Since I was sitting directly behind Mr Cai I was witness to the whole affair. The driver's face lit up. I could partly understand the exchange between him and Mr Cai. The driver had found a supplement to his food supply and knew that his family would be pleased about the event. For him it was a godsend. Cai nodded in our direction. We wouldn't understand this as doctors in the West, he said to the clearly disappointed man. In Europe this kind of thing wouldn't be understood in countries where dogs are kept, loved and protected as pets. The driver had tears in his eyes.

'My family is hungry,' said he.

Cai laid his hand on the man's shoulder and made it quite clear to him that he should leave the dog at the side of the road. Blood was still running from its snout. The deeply disappointed driver hesitated for some time before accepting the suggestion. Then he flung the hapless animal into the bush. Its coat was shiny, if unkempt, and the dog was large and healthy. It would have made a good meal. Chinese enjoy dog meat very much and like to eat it in the cooler season. Moreover, the dog, so to speak, is a mainstay in the prerequisites of the traditional apothecary, a kind of Chinese medicament.

As we got under way again, the driver did not sing any more and he drove much slower. I could see that he was still crying, and the tears were still running down his cheeks. No doubt he was thinking of the dead dog lying there to waste in the bush, and of the potential meal that had been denied him and his hungry family.

Once at the Ming graves, we all filed out of the bus and walked the long aisles between the grave mounds. The exercise in fresh air did us all good. In the empty tombs which had been plundered centuries before, it was pleasantly cool.

Haubensack informed us that in order to keep the location and the building techniques a secret, all the labourers taking part in the erection of the tombs were executed by imperial civil servants and soldiers after the work had been completed. Later, shallow graves were scratched in the soil for them not far away. Dr Cai knew his history and confirmed what Haubensack had related.

'So human life didn't count for much in ancient China,' said Adrienne. 'It makes me wonder they invented a form of medicine at all.'

Later on, we were driven to the Great Wall. This immense structure was erected in the years between AD 500 and 1200. It was built to keep out the continuous raids from hordes of Mongol marauders. There were soldiers dressed in the green uniforms of the Liberation Army with their red starred caps to be seen everywhere. They watched us with suspicion out of the corner of their eyes as if we were about to break a stone from the wall and take it home to Europe as a souvenir. Neither were they at all pleased about our taking photos.

This long, monumental ribbon of crenulated stone has a broad path at the top, and together we covered about a kilometre along its length. On the way, our Dutch colleague, Alice, wanted to know more about the dog incident; she had sat right at the back of the bus and didn't know the details.

'So the bus driver's family has to go hungry?'

'Here, everybody's hungry,' I said, 'and we'll be hungry ourselves before long.'

'This Cai's an inhuman fellow!' she said. 'And he actually justified his order not to take the dog home to eat because we might not approve?'

'Perhaps he would have liked to eat something of the dog himself, but didn't trust himself to say anything in front of us!'

'How brutal!' Alice said indignantly. 'It's all the damn same to me whether a Chinese eats a dog with relish or not, but I'm sorry when it comes to it that a family hasn't got enough on the table.'

'The Chinese don't understand us Europeans. Above all, they want to keep their noses clean. Don't lose face! That's the main thing. The last thing they want is that Europeans go around telling each other that the Chinese are dog-eaters. This, despite the fact that they all love dog meat. They even go hungry to save face.'

Dr Haubensack had caught up with us. 'This business with the dog is ridiculous,' he averred. 'A lot of daft folks here. At least I've learned that much. I had imagined China to be quite different.'

The huge watchtowers set at intervals along the famous wall as it ran over hill and dale seemed to be an endless chain of stone. Its course was finally lost in the misty infinity of the late afternoon. I ascended the steps at the side of the wall which led up to the parapet, first towards the east and then to the west. This gigantic construction of brick is over six hundred miles long and the astronauts tell us that it can even be seen from the moon.

'Ugh! The thickest wall is in the heads of the Chinese,' Haubensack commented as he sweated with effort at my side.

'Or in our own heads, perhaps.'

'We have to break through this wall', he insisted.

'Perhaps we can pierce it with an acupuncture needle?'

'That's got to be a huge needle.'

'Or with Chinese characters,' I mused.

'Could be,' he replied. 'By the way, could you teach me a few of these funny cryptograms, you think?'

'In Shanghai we'll have time for that,' I said.

II

Shanghai's 'Big Ben'

Today we arrived in Shanghai. Our dwelling for the next weeks would be in the Shanghai Da-Shan hotel in a brown rectangular tower located on the banks of the Su-Zhou Canal not far from the river Huang-Pu and close to the harbour. The hotel was erected by the British in the '20s. It was built on a cross-like foundation and was terraced so that every storey had a generous balcony. The hotel roof had a garden from where one could enjoy a view over the whole city, its harbour and the river below. Buildings of this kind, which originated in the first thirty years of the twentieth century, came into being in western cities first but could not be built by the Chinese architects at the time.

The wide, high windows were arranged in three wings, each wing having three thick panes secured in wrought-iron frames against rain and typhoons. On looking out, I could see the half-moon-shaped river promenade called 'The Bund'. Here, too, were other buildings constructed by Europeans which by now had lost some of their earlier gloss: banks in sugar-cake style, for example, former port authority offices, hotels and business houses. We found ourselves in fact in the former colonial centre of Shanghai.

An old bridge built along the lines of ancient Chinese architecture connected us with the city centre over a side stream of the Huang-Pu. The streets were lined with trees in fresh green foliage, and a small park on the banks of the river was situated at the entrance of the harbour where we could see smaller vessels anchored close together in groups. Further out, we could see larger freighters and a multi-deck ferryboat sailing slowly by. Between these vessels were dark wooden junks, their sails set, and among these all kinds of other boats from small to very small, some of them of the most outlandish construction, but all of them having one thing in common along with the Chinese national flag – namely, washing. On every vessel, washing was hung out to dry. On the water we could hear constant signals of varying kinds, from the reverberating boom of ocean liners to the squeaky hooting of ferryboats and the bell-like tinkling of smaller craft. The human voice blared through megaphones, bellowing orders or warnings into the environment. There was a lot going on. It was not for nothing that Shanghai had been dubbed 'the city on top of the sea'.

A hundred years ago, or only fifty, this harbour was even busier. That was in Shanghai's heyday at a time when western trading tycoons and investors set the pace. Many areas of China were under western influence at that time.

Dr Haubensack and I discovered that we would still be sharing the same room number. We found ourselves again in one single apartment, and so we demanded the promised separate rooms from our hosts, but this was like talking to a wall.

'We were assured of separate apartments when we were in Beijing,' we argued. 'After all, we're of a different nationality.'

'What goes for Beijing isn't true of Shanghai,' was the retort.

'Our states were hostile to one another for hundreds of years,' Haubensack persisted.

'Our fathers and grandfathers fought against one another in the last world wars!' added I.

This, apparently, was of no interest to the Chinese we had to deal with at that moment.

'And we can't stand each other; we hate each other!' Haubensack roared.

'That's of no concern to us', the official said coldly.

'Dr Haubensack speaks German and you, too, so you can get along with one another.' The party officals were adamant.

'I snore like a circular saw,' Haubensack added with emphasis, pushing his point. And I underlined this fact by adding that because of this I couldn't sleep a wink.

'It's unbearable! No one can sleep because of this snoring. Our German colleague could well fall ill for lack of sleep and you would be directly responsible. Indeed, my wife wanted to divorce me for it.'

'What does that mean, "divorce"?' the organiser enquired.

'This means when a man or a woman goes to court to apply for the dissolution of their marriage,' Haubensack explained.

'We've got nothing like that here,' the Chinese replied laconically, unperturbed by such a tragic possibility. 'With us, a man and a woman remain together for as long as they live when they're married.'

'Even if they can't stand the sight of one another and hate each other like poison … ?'

'As well,' the host replied.

'God! How awful!' Haubensack hissed. But nothing helped.

'You're together and that's it,' the man said.

Saying nothing to one another, we went up to our apartment.

'Perhaps we should catch the next plane back home,' I queried. My room companion sat there with a sullen expression and said not a word.

The clock over Shanghai's harbour struck midday, slowly, twelve times, its sound metallic, resonant, stirring, like that of a Tibetan gong. It was a souvenir from the British raj and its sound reminded one forcefully of London's 'Big Ben', whose tones, admittedly, are much softer, more sophisticated, and altogether nobler than this timekeeper. The British are not remembered here with much affection, and the Russians and the Americans with even less. This may well have to do with the Opium Wars in the nineteenth century. Hong Kong at that time was incorporated into the British Empire as a colony and grew to become the largest port in the Far East after English gunboats had sailed up the Pearl River and the inhabitants of many country provinces in China been forced to smoke their imported opium. Hong Kong and its English administration had always pleased me, and I valued the reliable order the city enjoyed and that was kept alive by colonial civil servants. I had worked there once as a doctor for a short time. However, I could not mention that here.

It was in Hong Kong that I made my first acquaintance with Chinese medicine. I received Chen-chiu treatment at the hands of an old man then, and afterwards I felt better than I had ever felt in my life before. For the first time I actually realised what health and well-being were. It was odd: I had studied medicine for six years, had worked as a medical man, had come across many patients and treated many, and yet, on the other hand, had never experienced such good health prior to that occasion.

Colleagues from the English Hospital had first sent me to this friendly individual with a beard over a foot long and consisting of about thirty strands of hair, some brown, some grey and some white. 'When we can't get any further with patients, we send them to him. He is always in a position to help somehow,' my Hong Kong colleagues said.

His place in Kowloon was the simplest set-up imaginable. He practised his art in a blue linen smock and with bare feet in sandals. He knew that I was a western doctor interested in Chinese medicine.

'If you really want to know what Chinese medicine is all about, you will have to go to mainland China', he said. He would say 'Da-Lu', as the Chinese call red China. 'The best places are either Beijing or Shanghai. Shanghai is the better known for its Chen-chiu specialists.' That was five years ago.

At that time I used to write articles for German newspapers on medical matters in the Far East. Among other things, I had been encouraged to write a highly critical article on the backwardness of Chinese medicine and acupuncture and, if possible, make it sound ridiculous. In Germany, people had an entirely wrong view of the concept of the Chinese capability to cure, and that originally included me.

Notwithstanding, I decided at that time to look into the matter more carefully and to actually try and discover what this curious and yet enthralling art of healing was about. The Chinese mainland, Da-Lu, was entirely cut off to foreigners at the time. An English businessman took me for a day once to a fair in Canton. I recall the journey as one beleaguered by police, military personnel and customs controls. Getting to know Chinese medical practitioners was quite out of the question.

'So they've decided after all to shove us together! What are we going to do, then?' my room companion demanded, 'Do we stay or do we go?'

Thinking of the difficulties associated with learning acupuncture and Chinese medicine in Europe, I said outright: 'We should stay.'

'Good. Then I'll stay on, too,' said Haubensack. 'And because I'm the oldest, I suggest we get along from now on with forenames. My name is Achille.'

'My name's Ralf Robert – Ralf for short,' I smiled.

I reminded myself of the fact that the use of a first name in French convention did not necessarily imply the corresponding use of the familiar form 'tu' (in German 'du'). That meant that I didn't automatically have the right to use this form with my companion. That would have meant a higher rung in the ladder of familiarity. We could not be said to know each other well enough for that, so we tacitly agreed to keep the formal address.

'And as far as your snoring goes, I can have a pair of earplugs sent over by airmail. Your thunder won't be so terrible then!'

I had found out that this kind of 'noise protection' was not available in China, perhaps because the Chinese are fond of every kind of noise. In order, it seemed, to emphasise just this point, an ocean-going liner was at that moment steaming down river below our window with the siren at full blast, a diapason so deep and vibrant that the panes in the windows shuddered in unison. In comparison with this, Haubensack's snoring was a mere twitter. I could forget a midday nap. I went into the bathroom, where I discovered that the first job was to shoo away a number of cockroaches. Hotel Da-Shan was an old establishment and as such was as delightful a place to settle in for cockroaches as an old ship.

After this informal introduction, we began to talk about medical matters.

Achille was of the opinion that 'if this business of acupuncture actually works – and this we will soon see – then it has to work as well in the West. And then it has to be brought into line with a western theory and explained in terms of that theory. If not, then the whole thing remains mere "suggestion" and we can forget it.'

He went on to say that if it functioned at all, then it was at the same time necessary to translate the Chinese texts properly into western languages and leave the Chinese out of the game once and for all. As a medical practitioner, one should not get involved in philological niceties. Perhaps he was right. He said that it was a matter of complete indifference as to whether this or that was called a 'point' or a 'meridian' or something else. The main thing was that from these 'points' and therapeutical rules one could produce something of medical utility.

I replied to all this by explaining that the old Chinese system of curing patients was deduced from the concepts of Yin and Yang and the Five Elements, as well as from coldness, heat, fire, emptiness, fullness, and understanding the superficial and interior aspects of the organism and filling up and reducing bodily functions, and that these ideas must first be thoroughly understood so that one could at all correctly carry out the therapies connected with them. The ensuing technique, after all, is the prerequisite for the efficacy of acupuncture.

'Very well,' he said, 'but finally we can certainly find a theory in western terms to account for its effectiveness. I'm convinced of this one thing: our objective must be to set up a correspondence between ancient Chinese medicine and modern western medicine and so optimise the potential of both.'

What Shall We Do With Our Libido?

We began to think again about what to do with our free evenings, whether or not we could find a pretty Chinese girl with whom we could spend an evening out. One of our female interpreters was very nice, for example. Today, for instance, a number of good-looking young women gave us the glad eye while we were in town. They turned round to look at us as we passed, and a few of them even winked at us. Shanghai in this respect is much more relaxed, more pleasant and open-minded than Beijing.

We visited the Seamen's Club where, to our consternation, we found, instead of attractive women, a horde of language students who assailed us with their broken English and tried to get us into conversation. In a bookshop I bought a large map of the country, while Achille bought an acupuncture chart in English, which had been published in China. Back in the hotel room he brought out a poster from *Playboy* of a naked brown-eyed blonde with large, voluptuous breasts. This he hung up on the wall of the hotel room. 'I've brought this along as a precautionary measure, so to speak, so that at least we have something female not far away,' he said.

Two female interpreters came once more to the room late in the evening. After noticing the *Playboy* poster and blushing to their ears with embarrassment, they didn't give it another glance. Nevertheless, they nudged each other and winked slyly. I remembered on my first visit to the Shanghai Academy of Medicine a little over three years ago that a doctor there wanted to confiscate the latest edition of *Der Spiegel* which I had with me. He indignantly explained that the magazine was a 'pornographic publication', because it displayed naked women and for that reason was forbidden in China.

'How do you know that, then?' I asked him. Presumably he had often seen the magazine before, but he wouldn't admit it. He went on about such things as this that in any case are forbidden to bring into a Chinese clinic and said that, for this reason, it must be confiscated immediately and destroyed. I gave it to him reluctantly and knew at the same time that long before the magazine's destruction it would do the rounds among the doctors. Chinese doctors, naturally, had to know what went on inside the heads of western physicians!

The two young women wanted the written text of my welcoming speech in French that was to be given at the College of Chinese Medicine tomorrow afternoon. They said that they needed the French text so that they could properly prepare a Chinese translation and not make a fool of themselves on the next day. During this encounter they giggled constantly, and, their faces still red to the ears, clumsily took their leave – not, however, without looking long and intensively at the poster!

I wrote up my speech and took it to the interpreters' room. Later, in the corridor, I met the senior interpreter, Old Lu, and talked to him briefly about Tai-Ji-Quan and Qi-Gong – Chinese gymnastics and health conditioning. When I said that, as a good Chinese doctor, one didn't actually heal just particular illnesses, but was obliged to get down to considering the background of a disease and so prevent its further development, he agreed. Actually curing just a disease is only the second step of a Chinese doctor. I suggested that it might be a good idea to organise an introductory course in Qi-Gong or Tai-Ji-Quan for us, and he agreed to do this.

At night there was a terrible row to be heard on the river and in the streets below the hotel. High women's voices screamed out revolutionary ballads in which Mao and the party were glorified, and these were accompanied by the most primitive orchestrations. I lay in my bed in a kind of half sleep. At around two in the morning the noise did abate somewhat for a couple of hours, only to begin again at five to the tune of ships' sirens, the hooting of cars and megaphones at full amplitude. At six, Shanghai's 'Big Ben' struck the hour, making the hotel windows shiver and rousing us all out of sleep. Everyone in Shanghai gets up at this time. The previous day I ordered ear plugs from Germany by telephone which would be sent by airmail. I just had to sleep somehow. I recalled the Chinese method of torture by which a prisoner was bombarded with high-pitched noise until he finally lost his mind and subsequently died.

And by the way, I have also to report on the day of my official welcoming speech at the institute and the honours and festivities connected with our arrival in Shanghai. In the morning, we had been treated to a city bus tour where we got to know only a little about the town. We were invited, for example, into the so-called Friendship Store, where the ordinary Chinese had no business to be and which was only for foreigners. Prices were higher than in other parts of the city, but there was a greater selection of usable goods.

From there we drove through this traffic-ridden metropolis, although there were few cars to be seen and a number of trucks. The greater part of the traffic consisted of cyclists. The bikes were all clean and polished and in best working order. They fulfilled their purpose in the same way a private car does in Europe. They were a status symbol. Some of the cyclists even wore white gloves. The road surface in the main arteries of the city was of asphalt and in good condition. In the smaller lanes off the main thoroughfares the surface was damaged, rough and uneven. Above many streets there were strings of telephone lines and the simplest light-bulb wires hanging into the road. Between the houses, washing swung from cords strung to the buildings. On some buildings there was scaffolding constructed of bamboo ready for further construction or for adding another storey. The workers operating on these unsteady structures had to have ape-like adroitness in order to keep their balance.

The unusual architecture of one building in an adjacent street caught my eye. I recognised it by its gothic pointed archway as a church entrance. Its former portal was constructed of dark, clinkered brick and had later been walled up. Crude red-brown wooden windows had been subsequently set in the concrete and from the whole hung hundreds of naked light bulbs on a horizontally stretched cable. At one time it had been a church, but it now functioned under socialism as a store for provisions. Today, it would be pitch black inside. The Communist Party was frightened to death by Christianity, by western philosophy, by Buddhism, and indeed by all kinds of ideology and congregational belief. Why? Because Maoist communism is itself an ideology. Mao had said that religion was poison for the people. In the country before his time, western missionaries had a pretty free hand in disseminating their ideas while along with them the greater part of the population was Buddhist. There were also a few Muslims here and there. Indeed, it was possible for one person to be a member of several religions, so that they could be a Christian, a Buddhist, a Taoist and a Muslim all in one. The Chinese have always been a careful people and one could never be sure what would happen after death! However, this disturbed the current party concept, in which Mao Tse-tung was the only recognisable 'god'.

At midday we were back at the hotel so that we could eat on time.

Before the actual event took place, everyone – that is, the professors, the teachers and their assistants – all greeted us on the steps of the academy with a handshake. Then we all proceeded into the main hall of the building where such celebrations usually take place. The chairman for cultural affairs in the city was present and it was he that then initiated proceedings. During his speech he mentioned the good relations enjoyed between our respective countries. One group of counter revolutionists was cited for stiff criticism again and again. It was referred to as the 'Gang of Four', which included Mao's wife, Lin Piao and Liao Shuo-Shi. Above all, Confucius came in for the harshest criticism of all and, in his opinion, ranked as China's worst ideological criminal in the whole of that country's history.

He went on to enumerate China's great achievements, especially the progress made under the administration of the new president of the party, Hua Kuo-Feng. 'Progress' is one of the most frequently used words here, but where, actually, is this progress to lead the state? Is it to become more and more orientated to the West and thereby introduce capitalistic structures? Here, one can talk to no one about that subject.

The places of honour were at the front of the hall, and the seats were occupied by the professors of the college, the representatives of the city, and those members of the Revolutionary Committee belonging to the academy in matters of traditional Chinese medicine. A row of speeches now began. The first to speak was the chairman of the Cultural Committee, then came the chairman of the Revolutionary Committee of the academy, followed by our host from the Beijing Ministry of Health, Dr Cai, who was followed in turn by the Director of the Shanghai Ministry of Health. All of them said essentially the same thing and one had the feeling that one speaker could be randomly exchanged for the next without anyone noticing. People with their own personal flair and style are just not on the agenda of public affairs here.

After these formal introductions were over, it was my turn. The French term for 'Germany' is 'Allemagne' and this begins with 'A', the first letter of the alphabet. That was why I had to begin. After me came the men from Cameroon and Chad, then the French folks, the representatives of the Netherlands, and so on. For my part, I read every word from the script. The same applied to the other national representatives. Our Chinese hosts were thanked in politely formal terms for the invitation to China and the hope was expressed for a consolidation of good relations in the future between China and the countries present. When we had all said our piece, there was a declaration over a loudspeaker: The ceremony was at an end. Everyone immediately stood up and returned to his or her respective omnibus. I had the feeling that nothing had actually happened. Stand up, speak up and shut up, every speech calculated to say nothing. During the event there was any amount of green tea to drink, poured out for us by young Chinese women who, for the length of the whole proceedings, held their eyes down in an attitude of ashamed humility.

After we had returned to the hotel, Achille and I decided to walk a little along The Bund. The banks along it were still open and I decided to go into one of them, and so went up to the cash desk and found to my astonishment that I could easily exchange my traveller's cheques without the slightest inconvenience – the same cheques that I had wanted to change in Beijing, where I was assured that I would not be able to change them anywhere in China. Everything here was easier going than in Beijing. This could be seen in the way women and girls greeted us and waved to us on the street, a gesture which was to be interpreted as an amicable greeting to China's friends. Perhaps it meant more, who knows? I say this because sometimes they remained standing and looked at us in a soliciting way, so that one could assume that they wanted to talk to us. From time to time I asked them their names, which they were always willing to tell me. Then I told them my Chinese name and they were greatly amused.

One asked, 'How is it that you have a Chinese name?'

I told them that this name was given to me by a Chinese interpreter some years ago. This caused uproarious laughter all round. Chinese often laugh not because they are amused, but because they are embarrassed.

Lovers were often seen here wrapped up in each other in the parks. That too was different from the capital of workers, civil servants and soldiers, Beijing.

A few minutes before seven in the evening, there was a knock on the door. It was one of our interpreters who had come to warn us please to be prompt for the evening meal. Apparently, it annoyed them, our easy-going, European manner. We would have to be initiated into the drill and discipline of a socialist state. In this place, everyone was politically matter-of-fact, punctual; everyone gave one the impression that he or she was responsible for the whole apparatus, and this is something which Europeans just don't go for.

The evening banquet to mark the occasion of our initiation into the secrets of Chinese medicine took place in the banqueting hall of Shanghai Da-Shan, in the same building that housed our hotel room. The tables were decorated with large turntables, so-called Lazy Susans on which could be found the most delicious of Chinese delicatessen specialities. Next to every place at dinner were several glasses, one for wine, one for beer and one for schnapps. Once more according to the order of the western alphabet I was placed to the right of the representative of the Ministry of Health, and to my right sat the chairman for cultural affairs, and this position happened by chance to be the most honourable in the hierarchical order of rank. However, here it simply meant the order of the alphabet.

By this arrangement, then, I found myself sitting with the most distinguished guests – among others, the oldest professor for medicine at the academy. At our table were those who had been in China for the second or third time. As I said above, these were referred to by the Chinese as 'old friends'. Among these was the doctor from Cameroon, Adnan Kirinin, about whom Haubensack had remarked that 'he smokes his cigarettes like a chimpanzee'. This African colleague also spoke some Chinese, and did so by pursing his lips, his face radiant with goodwill. He was doing just that in conversation with a bald-headed Chinese professor whose name I've forgotten.

Adrienne Coningk, the blonde, beautiful young woman from Holland who had a very determined air about her, delivered an excellent speech in French. Her forefathers came from France and she was the only one from our motley crew this evening who was obliged to speak at table. A number of us had already aired the opinion that we were treated more like students here, with all the advantages and disadvantages this condition carries. Some of us – one noted – were already inclined to provocation, the cheeky aside and the practical joke. I would never have thought that twenty years after my last year at school I would be submitted to this kind of regimen again.

Dr Kang and I carried on a conversation across the table on the various effects needle and moxa therapy have on westerners and Chinese. It was generally agreed that anatomically and psychologically there was no difference and that they were quite the same. However, I said, I had found that a man living in the West under the capitalist dispensation has to undergo more stress than the Chinese. The difference in the two political systems could have an influence on the effects of these therapies, in either a positive or a negative sense. However, politics, we quickly agreed, was a theme we should not touch upon this evening. Our hosts gently changed the subject.

Everything was plentiful and of high quality and served by pretty waitresses, and I thanked Dr Cai, who was sitting on my left, for this kind hospitality. He replied that, yes, this was so. 'We offer our guests the best we have, but we don't eat like this every day, as you will no doubt learn as you go on.'

We tried to eat with our chopsticks so well that we could take up a peanut with them. 'Is that a kind of a practical entrance examination?' I asked. 'It's certainly a good exercise for the fingers and so useful for the practice of acupuncture.'

Dr Kang was amused by this and agreed wholeheartedly. 'Have you done a lot of acupuncture in Germany?' he asked, and I told him that I had an average of about twenty or thirty patients a day.

'Exactly the same number as I have,' he said, astonished. That our top acupuncturists in Europe have reached almost the same standards of accomplishment as the practitioners here I declined to say of course.

At the end of the meal, the chairman of the Revolutionary Committee stood up, raised his glass, and came round to each one of us. We in turn raised ours with a 'Gan-Bei', which literally means 'The dry glass!' or 'To the bottom of the vessel.' We toasted each individual in the group. We used to refer to this as 'Ex' in German students' groups and fencing schools. On such occasions one had to be able to hold one's liquor, my goodness!

Schnapps followed. This was called Mao-Tai, and it went straight to the bones and head. It was pretty cheap stuff and had a peculiar, synthetic smell. It was the kind of thing used to clean rusty hinges or remove the layers of dirt from door handles. No one in Europe would think of actually drinking it. Notwithstanding, we were all to raise our glasses and drink to our interpreters. The dinner lasted exactly two hours. That, we were to understand, was that.

No one lingered to talk. There were no pleasantries as is customary in Europe on such occasions. Everyone hurried to the door where our host, a representative of the city of Shanghai, stood to shake our hands once more.

'Xien-Cai Xiu-Xi,' he said in farewell. This means, in so many words, 'Now, if you don't mind, we'll all go to bed and sleep.'

That was all very well, but would it be possible to sleep with all that hullabaloo outside? Achille and I were of the same opinion: the answer was 'No'. So we went on a little footwalk together down the Huang-Po and back on the main road.

A Shanghai Clochard

We wandered over the railway bridge and along the river and took Nanjing Street into the city. On the way a strange type crossed our path, an old, bearded individual in rags, with a battered straw hat on his shorn head and carrying an army hip flask. He was unsteady on his feet and reeked of alcohol. So there are these types here as well, we concluded. Was he really an alcoholic? Amazed, we asked ourselves whether he was perhaps the Chinese variety of the French clochard, the kind one sees in Paris.

He seemed to understand what we were saying to each other, and then suddenly he asked: 'Hey! Spreshen Sie Deutsch?'

We spoke to him in German and immediately we were bombarded with a hail of German expressions. He was 56 years old, he told us, and formerly a seaman who had sailed on many a German ship. He was glad to see us, he said, 'so nice to shpreshen Deutsch again'.

Then he fell into English and told us that he also spoke English. 'I shpeak French, too,' he added, 'I shpeak everything.'

Because he could speak other languages, he was at one time employed at the Shanghai Seaman's Club, he went on to tell us, and he had just come from there. He worked in a foundry for a living. Apparently, his good relations with the Seaman's Club had allowed him to fill his flask with schnapps.

We asked him whether we could pick up a couple of pretty girls in the neighbourhood. He looked at us with his tragic Chinese brown eyes and I noticed the thick circle of ageing greyness around the pupils. He pulled Achille by the sleeve and murmured something almost to himself.

'Oh, boys, you are forty years late!' he said.

'Yes! And that's our opinion too,' remarked Achille.

'At one time here, there was plenty, plenty! Wonderful Chinese women. That's all gone, now. Pity. Prostitution has all gone. Cleaned out. Pity. Great pity!'

For Achille, the mention of 'prostitution' grated.

'Another shitty bourgeois tag that these communists have taken up in the same way as those damned moralists in Europe do to spoil the best thing in the world. Trust them to drag it through their muck and then ban it as something disgusting,' he said.

'You should only have intercourse with your wedded wife or with a partner you've agreed to live with,' I replied.

'And if that's not possible?' Achille asked.

'Then you have to think of something; there's always a way.'

'And that bearing in mind that Mao has torn 'heart' 心 out of the character "love".'

The clochard tottered along in front, obviously pleased that he could speak to us.

Achille asked him how he felt living in China.

'Oh, not so bad. I have everything I really need,' he answered in a manner that would lead us away from the topic. It seemed that he received enough booze to keep him going. After all, he was clearly an alcoholic.

We went along with him for a while. He reeled from time to time and kept repeating: 'Oh boys, oh boys ...'

Then he suddenly turned to me and said in German, 'Mein lieber Mann! [Oh, my good man!]'

We wanted to invite him to some place to have a short drink. He would certainly have a lot of interesting things to tell us. But it was about a quarter past eleven and everything would be closed. No restaurants, no bars, no place in the whole of Shanghai was open at this time of night – not even one of the many eating houses along the streets would be there to offer us a morsel or two, and that in a metropolis of several million inhabitants. Thirteen million people live in this city, a place larger than London and the largest city in the whole of the Chinese republic. The town was dead.

'Where shall we go?' we asked ourselves, and just kept walking ahead along the street called The Bund, a prohibited area for the Chinese and open only to foreigners in the past. At one time there was an infamous sign here in the park which warned: 'CLOSED TO DOGS AND CHINESE'.

This kind of thing had a lasting effect on the population at large and lingers in its collective memory. Westerners were and still are the 'devils from overseas'.

We said goodbye to our companion – our clochard, as we had dubbed him – at a rather dark corner. Indeed, this old seaman did look like the kind of tramp that can be seen in Paris. We would not have encountered such a person in Beijing.

Back at the hotel, we engaged in another long talk about the theory of Chinese medicine. Achille repeated his view that it was enough to observe the effects of treatment and just copy it. One could do without a theory for the time being. It was sufficient merely to study the effects of application, but we would have to get to know them carefully. As for operating techniques: when we had applied these sufficiently often, we would be able to do them in our sleep and then there would be no need for theory. I answered to the effect that the theory of needle therapy depended on a thousand years of experience and was sensible in so far as it was based on the relevant observations made of nature. These can still be used today. Why should one just throw all this overboard?

Achille did not agree with me. He felt that I was a typical German philosopher, a head-type kind of person. As such a type, I would naturally enjoy the theory more than the practice. This, however, was not true. I myself am also an ardent practitioner, but I like to discuss things, that I must own.

The next night was quieter; there was not so much external noise and sleep was only occasionally disturbed by Achille's snoring. The tooting of steamers coming and going in the harbour, which in any case was the same day and night, was from time to time interrupted by the loud hooting of ships' sirens. Was it also a fact that we were getting used to it all? After a while here, Shanghai no longer gives one the impression of being a large metropolis. It has something of the idyllic and rural about it, almost as if it were a large village. We slept better and deeper until the next morning.

During the day, there was a broad view of the park from the hotel window. This was the park that was once forbidden to dogs and Chinese. At this time of the morning, people could be seen practising Qi-Gong and Tai-Ji-Quan and one could encounter parents on walks with their progeny until late in the evening. An old man sat in a pavilion with a younger man showing him how to play the two-stringed fiddle, the Er-Hu. A few sat pondering moves in a game of chess. Everything was composed, quiet and relaxed. It was the opposite indeed to our own hectic western way of life where people fearfully isolate themselves from others. Here, there was a chance to speak to one another, to express happiness, even if this only meant waving at each another. In this way at least I felt that this community had something to offer which was of human value.

I walked alone along Nanjing Street, where I had discovered a shop displaying paper, writing materials, coloured pencils and pens, and also a Chinese brush. I went in.

'Mao-bi you mei you?' I asked. 'Have you a brush to write Chinese characters?'

The saleswoman did not understand at first what I wanted. For her, I sounded strange, partly I am sure because my Mandarin pronunciation was not something she was in daily contact with as her customers spoke Shanghai dialect. So I repeated my request.

'I would like a "mao-bi", a writing brush,' and so saying, I pulled at my hair so as to show her what I meant and repeated the word, 毛, mao, hair.

This she understood and said, 'Do you know, I've been selling these brushes for twenty years, but have never associated the term mao with hair!

You're the first person to draw my attention to it. I just say the words mechanically and think no more about it. Many thanks!'

Did all Chinese treat their written and spoken language with the same indifference? I purchased a number of brushes, some large sheets of white paper and black ink. On the way back to the hotel I began thinking about what the woman had said. It became clear to me on the way that the reason the Chinese so seldom pause to reflect on what their characters really mean and the reason they are not usually in a position to explain them is because have never learned how they are made up from their components. They use their characters mechanically without reference to their inner logic.

On my return to the hotel I mentioned this to Achille, who was as surprised about this fact as I was and who was also pleased about the present of brush and paper I had with me for him.

We Start Studying Acupuncture

Today was our first day of instruction at the Shang-Hai Zhong-Yi Xue-Yuan, the Shanghai College of Chinese Medicine. One can variously translate the term for 'college' as 'institute' or 'academy'. More recently, the academy has begun to use the title Shang-Hai Zhong-Yi Da-Xue, the University for Chinese Medicine. This title came into being as the result of the need to raise its status for international cooperation. A university enjoys more kudos than perhaps a college does. Despite this, the same teachers and the same material make up the faculty; it is run on the same principles as before.

The morning was taken up with informing us about the Chinese health system as practised in Shanghai. It was emphasised that one of the main objectives was to combine traditional Chinese medicine with that of the West. It was clear that one will not get far in the modern world relying on Chinese traditional methods alone. According to the information given to us, there are 393 hospitals in the city – that is to say, 47,794 beds, with 13,000 medical technicians employed. Eleven thousand doctors with western training work here, together with 4,822 traditionally trained Chinese doctors. On average, both groups of doctors go through a six-year training period. To their number another group of doctors can be added who only do a three-year period of training. This group comprises 13,197 doctors, and altogether there are 21,539 nurses.

The College of Chinese Medicine was founded in 1956, with a study period of six years. At the time I was there, there were 120 students. For some time by then there had been a facility for doctors qualified in western medicine wanting to further their studies in Chinese medicine. This period of further study covers another two years, and at that time comprised 70 doctors.

Since the Cultural Revolution, the period of study has been reduced from six to three years. This was deemed necessary in order to train more doctors. Students are recruited from the ranks of farmers, workers and soldiers. People who had once been associated with former 'capitalist' families are barred from medical studies on principle.

I sat with Achille. Now and again when I looked at him as the lectures droned on, he shook his head. 'How the heck can you make a good doctor out of a Chinese farmer or a worker having no intellectual background?' he asked.

'They'll make as good a doctor as you'd get from a western farmer or worker,' I answered.

'We mustn't get ill while we're here,' he added, 'otherwise they'll quickly do us in, these farmers and workers.'

'We'll look out.'

I actually knew what he was talking about. On the other hand, I knew that in practice it was not as bad as we might imagine. I thought back to my first time as a stand-in at a practice in Germany. I had just qualified and was seconded to a rural practice in the Rhineland area. Here I had to face the task of dealing with an influenza epidemic and was soon in deep water. It is worth mentioning that at this time I had a six-year period of study behind me, had passed the examination well and written a good dissertation, and had spent half a year in surgery and a further six months in a gynaecology department, and a whole year studying and practising internal medicine under the guidance of a famous haematologist and another renowned nephrologist. In addition to this were my activities as a house surgeon in Britain and my time in Hong Kong, which were acknowledged as added experience during training. Yet, despite everything, I was unable to manage the treatment of a common or garden influenza epidemic. Highly qualified and yet totally incompetent in practice! Things like this are not uncommon in Germany. I asked myself at the time: 'What on earth did they teach you at those specialist clinics?'

When I was standing in as a locum for a colleague who was on holiday, and of course needed an assistant in the practice, it was a young receptionist who now stepped in to save the situation. She sent the best pharmaceutical representative who visited the practice in to me. This man, who was neither a doctor nor anything approaching it, recommended his firm's newest influenza medicaments and I shall always remain grateful to him. I busily applied his recommendations to my sick patients in the following two weeks and they proved to be salutary to the poor folks I had to deal with at that time.

My prominent teachers had only concerned themselves with research on and treatment of rare diseases, since this contributed to their international fame. How to treat a common cold did not appear on their teaching programmes as this didn't bring them any distinction. For this reason, those leaving their venerable teaching establishments were not equipped to deal with the challenges presented to general practitioners.

Is the situation any different in China?

Yes, perhaps these soldiers, these farmers and workers are better at managing day-to-day illnesses than the pedigree clinical consultants from western universities and the scientists of world repute.

And then there are people of whom one can say that they have the gift of healing 'in their blood' even if they have no scientific training whatsoever. Such were my reflections at this point, and I looked over to my companion for a reaction.

'Mon dieu,' he sighed, 'what next?'

Next came a lecture given by a thin, pale-faced party member and comrade with a gravelly voice and a sergeant major's manner, stuffed into a uniform with a high-fitting Mao collar. The lecture mainly consisted of vehement criticism of Confucius and, parallel to this, criticism of a certain Lin Piao whom no one would know of in ten years' time because he was so insignificant. However, here he had fallen into political disrepute and this made him interesting in a negative way. One or two Chinese professors on the rostrum yawned discreetly.

The great Confucius, referred to as Kung-tse in Chinese, was dragged through the dust of his lecturer's venomous tirade and I asked myself why. What cultural delusion so afflicted this individual that he could curse one of China's greatest teachers and speak of him now as a common rogue, a kind of criminal, this great man who, along with Lao-tse, did so much for the Chinese Empire – not to mention the Japanese and the Korean people? This deep aversion may well have come about during Mao's childhood, as his father, we are told, was a strict adherent of Confucius' teaching and frequently brought the unruly young Mao to task. In other words, the son later sought revenge on the worthy master, Kung, and presented him as a criminal active against China's morals. He did this to justify his own biographical background and to save his face. He was now in a position to do this, 'Sun King' of the China state that he was. Mao Tse-tung had in any case no desire to breed thinking, virtuous Chinese who honoured their parents, people who were able to read the great old books and understand them. All he wanted was a people comparable to blue ants, sexless machines who were only able to serve him and his party.

Later, we all assembled at the hotel again to eat. In the afternoon we received our first lesson in the 'History of Chinese Medicine', introduced by a short, very muscular professor who had something bucolic about him. He was a typical southern Chinese and his delivery was good. He was practically minded and his words were clearly backed up by much experience. He spoke about the origins of Chen-chiu some six thousand years ago, and about the discovery mentioned in the *Nei-Jing* that fire can heal and also about the nine classic needle types. He referred to the *Shen-Nung Ben-Cao-Jing*, the first classic work to deal with herbal medicine. He spoke of the physician Bian Que of the fourth century BC, who is accredited with the authorship of the *Nan-Jing*, the classic work on difficulties occurring when practising acupuncture. The *Huang-Di Nei-Jing* was mentioned on several occasions, this being a key work of reference on the subject up to the present time. The famous surgeon and acupuncturist Hua-Tuo, with his pain-reducing herbal remedy called Ma-Fei-San, was also alluded to in connection with the remedy's application during his famous risky operations on the human abdomen. The paravetertebral points which have been named after him were a matter of discussion, as well as his famous physical exercises imitating the movements of five animals: the tiger, the bear, the ape, the crane and the stag. He also referred with appreciation to Wang Fu-mi and his *Systematic Reference Book of Acupuncture and Moxibustion*, the first great methodical work in this specialist area, which appeared in the year AD 282. In addition to all this, the professor also alluded to Sun Si-miao, the author of *One Thousand Golden Prescriptions*, in which the technique of acupuncture is extensively treated. In conclusion, he did not fail to mention the fact that on its march through the country of more than 15,000 miles, the Red Army under Mao Tse-tung directly experienced the good results of traditional Chinese medicine, especially of acupuncture. Today, he concluded, the time has come for closer cooperation between western medicine and Chinese traditional medicine in the war against disease.

Bravo!

I noticed during the lecture that the text accompanying the illustrations that were used during it comprised a confusing mixture of the various ways of transposing the Chinese characters into their respective western counterparts – the Hanyu Pinyin, the Wade–Giles, together with the French Crivellier adoption as another example, were all used in a quite arbitrary way. As a consequence, chaos ensued. I had experienced this three years previously in the case of a Chinese man introducing hinself on his visiting cards as, say, Mr Huang, and on the next occasion as Mr Hoang and then later as Mr Wang, or even 'Wong'. The Chinese characters on the card, however, clearly gave the Chinese ideograph for 'yellow' – the man's actual name.

That day, following the lectures, Haubensack and I were punctually at table for dinner after having been late on the previous few occasions and reaping disapproval as a result. Neither of us was in any way a 'military type'. We took it easy in the apartment, lounged about and entered into long discussions on this and that.

On what? On virtually everything. Everything that took our fancy. Here, as time went on, we were requested in a friendly way to keep things tidy. One of the hotel boys remarked once in the lift during the afternoon that dinner would be served at 7 p.m., which, in our case, he went on, no doubt would mean that we'd turn up about half an hour later. The lad laughed to hide his embarrassment at saying such a thing.

'No,' we said, 'tonight we'll be there punctually at seven.'

For the Chinese, a meal is at the centre of the day's business, and as a result, one greets the other with a 'Chi Fan-le?' – 'Have you already eaten?'

That evening I found myself sitting next to Adnan, the doctor from Cameroon whose family name is 'Kirinin'. I figured that this was a name stemming from German colonial times in southwest Africa and was a derivative of the word 'klein', meaning 'small'. It may have been applied to his forefathers, indicating small stature, but it certainly did not apply to my huge, powerfully built table companion who even referred to himself as 'le Gorille', the Gorilla. The name, of course, could have once been used humorously to mean exactly the opposite! He frequently referred to himself in the third person, telling us what the 'Gorilla' had been doing during the day.

A Bet on Chinese Characters

On one of the following evenings, I conducted an experiment with Achille, who had continued talking about 'stupid Chinese characters'.

I furnished myself with writing materials, a brush, ink, a felt-tip pen and several large pieces of paper. Then I said: 'I'd like to make a bet with you.'

'A bet?'

'Yes, a bet on ten bottles of Qingdao beer.'

A little before I had stopped off at the bar and asked the bar team to reserve several bottles of beer for us each day.

'What's it all about, then?'

'I bet that you can write Chinese, Achille.'

'You'll lose.'

'Are you going to take me on?'

'Of course! You know how much I enjoy a glass of beer. After all, I'm an Alsatian!'

'Well,' I said. 'Then just forget all your academic, western learning. Try and be a boy of about five or six who hasn't gone to school yet.'

'That's not difficult,' he grinned.

'Good, and then you can write Chinese!'

'How can I?'

'Just as I say: you can quickly learn to write Chinese.'

'Ralf, my lad, you're joking!'

'No, not at all. Sit down, now, in front of the paper. That's right. Take the felt-tip pen and just write 1, 2 and 3 as a five-year-old would do.'

Achille then sat down and painted six vertical strokes. Between the first and the second and between the third and the fourth he left a small space, so that it looked like this: I II III. He looked up. 'Do you mean like this?'

'Exactly! Now turn the paper round clockwise at 90 degrees.'

He did so.

'Here you have the Chinese for "one", "two" and "three" written perfectly'

一

二

三

He looked blank. 'Is it so easy? The characters I've seen are much more complicated.'

'It only looks like that. The more complicated signs can be studied later. First of all, I have to say one or two things about the three signs you have already painted. The "one", 一, is pronounced "Yi" and stands for the One – namely, the whole of the universe. Two as depicted here is pronounced "Er", and it represents the "Yin" of Yin-Yang, which is the core of Chinese medicine. And the three, 三, "San", here is the "Yang". The two parallel lines of "two", 二, stand for the vulva of a female, the loins of a woman from which all life comes into being. The three strokes 三 are denoting "three" parts of the male genitals, two testicles and the penis. This has to do with sex and with reproduction as well.'

'They don't tell us anything about this at the academy,' Achille said.

'They know all about it, of course, but won't mention it because they're too cautious as they think we wouldn't understand.'

'So they keep certain things secret from us?'

'Quite a lot!'

'What a gang of false teachers!'

'The three strokes, 三, San, also mean the complete "world" in total. The heavens are above us, the human being is in the middle, and the earth is under our feet. If we connect all three strokes with a vertical one, 王, we have "king" or "emperor", Wang, 王. He has the task of maintaining harmony between heaven, human beings and the earth. That is the original Chinese world's order, to be achieved and to be maintained. Draw it, now.'

Achille painted the 'king', 王, Wang in Chinese, by connecting the three lines of 'three' with one single vertical line.

'So. In the last five minutes you've drawn four Chinese characters perfectly and correctly,' I said. 'That's quite an achievement.'

Achille was amazed.

'Now decorate the king with a costly jewel, which you can place at the bottom right, rendered simply as a short dot. This is the character 玉, Yu, and it means jade, which is a precious stone – in other words, a jewel that is fit for a king.'

Achille placed the dot in its right position.

'And now use your pen to box it in all the way round the whole so that it looks like a rectangle.'

He did so.

'That's called 国, Guo, a nation, a state, a valuable jewel within the country's borders. Your country, Achille, for example, is 法国, Fa-guo in Chinese characters, and mine is called 德国, De-guo. That we can have a look at later.'

'A rectangle means a country or a state, then?'

'Actually, it's called "the earth"; a circle, on the other hand, means the sky or heaven, ○. The rectangle with a vertical stroke through its middle denotes "China". You can write this, too, just a simple square, 口, and then draw a vertical stroke through the middle, 中, Zhong.'

Achille then did so, and the Chinese symbol for 'China', the 'centre', appeared.

'However, this symbol means much more. It implies the balance of human life, the "golden mean", for example, and also the "Middle Way" of Confucius which every Chinese should adopt in life according to the rules of the ancient teaching. This applies, too, in ancient Chinese medicine. So it's a very important character for us. If you now write the character for jade in the square and place that for China in front of it, then you have 中国, Zhong Guo, "China".'

'And you really think that the Chinese can read my scribble?' he asked.

'No doubt about it. We can prove it later by asking one of the interpreters to confirm what I say. If you like, you can write a few more characters so that the whole thing's worthwhile.'

Achille was motivated.

'Now just paint a man as children do, a line here and there to denote legs.'

He did so: 大.

'Much too complicated!' I objected. 'What's the most important thing about people?'

'The head.'

'Really? For us Europeans perhaps, but not for the Chinese.'

'It's not the genitals for sure, because we've already had these.'

'What then?'

'Legs, perhaps . . . ?'

'Correct! The human being is always on the go; so paint the legs.'

Achille then drew an 'up' and 'down' stroke, 人.

'There we are. He's standing there – or rather, he's on the way somewhere. He's called "ren", 人, the Chinese human being, a man.'

Achille wanted to write a whole lot more characters.

'Good. Now this human being wants to show us what "big" is. How do you think he can do that? What would a child do here?'

'He would stretch out his arms.'

'That's it.'

'So now we draw a horizontal line through the figure 'ren' to denote the idea of "large", "great": 大, "da" in Chinese.'

'That's simple', he commented.

'And the big "lid" placed over everything – what do we call that?'

'A lid?'

'Yes – what is the biggest "lid" for us human beings and the world?'

'The sky perhaps?'

'Right! Put in the sky or the heavens.'

Achille drew a horizontal line on top of the symbol for 'great' (da) 天 and looked at me, shaking his head.

'Perfect,' I said. 'That's called *tian*, heaven, the sky etc., but before you get tired, paint a woman – that's to say, a real woman here in desolate China!'

Achille drew a pointed triangle, a head and two legs.

'Much too complicated! What's the most important thing about a woman?'

He laughed.

'Now come on; you know.'

He painted a circle and grinned.

'Yes, well, but a bit more elegantly and much more in the abstract. The most important feature is the cavity in the woman's inside where the child can grow. Naturally, the legs are also important, but these are rather shorter in China than those of a man.'

'You'll have to show me that one,' Achille urged. 'Otherwise I'm sure to forget it again.'

'You were near.'

'I'll show you a Chinese woman,' I said, and I drew it for him, 女. 'It is pronounced nü.'

'It's important that you draw the lines in the right sequence, I'll show you that later. Now, paint the symbols one after the other with me.'

He did so.

'The Chinese knew about human beings, the world and women. If you paint two women, one above the other, then this might mean "pretty" or also deceitful, cunning or crafty. In Mandarin, it is pronounced "chiao", but in today's Pinyin transcript it is written as *jiao*.'

Achille drew two women, 妄, one above the other.

'Now paint three women as a pyramid, 姦. This means lasciviousness, rape, obscenity, or something indecent, a break in marriage. It's pronounced "*chien*" and in Pinyin spelled "*jien*".'

'Is that obscene enough?' asked he.

'That's quite good!' I said, delighted.

'A jolly game,' Achille enthused.

'You see, a real woman is always seen as only one good woman for the Chinese man. And for the right woman there must be a child. That's a stable situation and a firm tradition in China. Paint a child.'

Achille drew a wrapped-up child with outstretched arms.

'Even simpler.'

He painted the rough outline of a baby. 'Now divide that in half and put two arms on it.'

He painted the child, 子, '*zi*'.

'Now for cherry on top. If you're going to draw a woman and child, combining them like this, then that in Chinese is "good", 好, "hao". We hear this word all the time every day – hen hao, hao ma? bu hao, ni hao . . .'

Achille studied the symbol.

'Well now, just two other characters,' I said encouragingly. 'You remember "big", the man with outstretched arms? How, then, would you write "small"?'

Achille let both arms fall in his depiction. 'Like this perhaps?'

'Write that!' I demanded.

He drew the man on two legs with his arms hanging.

'Even simpler. It's enough now to depict the human being with one stroke and put two arms on each side of it.'

He wrote 小.

'That's right. This means "small": 小, "*xiao*", and it's pronounced "hsiao". It's used every day as well. "*Xiao zi*", 小子, are small children. One uses this word, 小, "*xiao*", to speak to young women and girls, *xiao jie*. Xiao followed by the family name is also used. Madame Gu is "Xiao Gu (Hsiao Ku)" in colloquial Chinese. *Xiao ren* (hsiao ren), 小人, on the other hand, means a "crafty person", a "little man", but in a contemptuous way.'

Achille listened attentively.

The very last character for today, and this one is derived from the idea of "small" and means "few" or "less". Beneath the hanging arms we can put a stroke like this: 少.'

Achille wrote the character.

'This is pronounced as "shao". It's also a character from acupuncture teaching. What Europeans call the "gall bladder meridian" is referred to in Chinese as "*shao Yang*" – "the smaller Yang". We'll get back to that one later. Suffice it to say now that "shao nü", 少女, is a young woman. This phrase is used to refer to our interpreters.'

'I've lost the bet,' said Achille sadly.

'Probably,' I replied. 'But on the other hand, you've had your first instruction in how to write sixteen Chinese characters, and that in less than half an hour.'

'Get the interpreters to come here,' Achille requested.

I went out into the corridor to see whether one of our helpers was near and came across one of them, our Hsiao Ku (Xiao Gu).

'Would you have a minute or two for us?' I asked courteously.

'Why?' she enquired with some suspicion.

'Please come over to our apartment.'

'To do that I will have to fetch a colleague. I'm not allowed to go to our guests' rooms on my own.'

She then went into the interpreters' office and asked for a fellow interpreter to come with her. It was Hsiao Chang. They were not very willing, but deigned to come with me.

'You've still got that indecent picture on the wall, haven't you?' enquired Hsiao Chang.

'I can take it down if it annoys you,' I said.

'No, no, no,' she stuttered, 'that won't be necessary.'

They then came into our room. Achille looked at his characters as though hypnotised. He handed his handwritten page to her.

'Please read this to us aloud,' he said.

Xiao Gu put on the most bored expression she could muster:

'I, er, san, wang, yu, da, tian, nü, chiao.' She pulled herself together for the next character and looked at us disapprovingly.

'Where did you get these bad characters?' She looked at the poster on the wall.

'Ah, I see,' she said. 'It's western decadence.'

'There's nothing like that in socialist China,' Xiao Chang confirmed.

Then Xiao Gu read on. 'Zi, hao, xiao, xiao zi, xiao ren, shao, shao nü ...'

'Can you read all that?' Achille had an expression of dubious amazement.

'Of course!' said Xiao Gu, putting down the paper. 'It's not a calligraphic piece of art, but it's correct Chinese. Why? Anyone can read it. Who wrote it, by the way?'

'I did,' Achille said, raising his head towards the ceiling.

Xiao Gu was speechless. In effect she said nothing in response, and that, for her, who was forever commenting on all that happened in rigid revolutionary terms, was a rarity. She even looked a little foolish. Clearly, she was about to lose face.

'Many thanks for your assistance, Ladies Gu and Chang,' I said. 'We'll see each other tomorrow in the clinic.'

Both of them left the room in haste, their eyes half closed. They would have to report this unbelievable piece of news to the Revolutionary Committee as soon as possible.

'Now I'm learning to write Chinese,' Achille said, pushing air through his lips in a kind of gasp, allowing himself to drop into an armchair. 'I tried to learn something at home about the language, at least the basics, but it was hopeless.'

'That was your teacher's fault,' I said.

'And I had lessons from a real Chinese woman, a tutor from the University of Nancy. She wrote her characters so quickly and in an illegible kind of handwriting that no one could decipher.'

'Chinese can very probably teach the spoken language, but they are hardly likely to be able to explain the inner logic of their written language,' I explained.

'Is Chinese logical at all, then?'

'Yes. It is based on the logic of painted pictogram. I think I mentioned this before in the plane. Every character has a logical structure.'

'I admit defeat. Now I've really lost the bet. Come, let's go downstairs to consume one of those ten bottles of Qingdao beer.' We went off.

'Do you think we could go on with this interesting game occasionally?' he asked when we had reached the restaurant.

'What else could we do here on our evenings?' I said.

'We could now actually call each other "tu" (French) or, in German, "du",' he proposed.

An Evening Stroll Through Shanghai

It had become a habit for us now to wander along the streets near the harbour. We tried to strike up conversation with one or two Chinese women, but they closed up, and when I asked them in Chinese whether they spoke English, they said not a word. The many passers-by, though, looked at us carefully. They actually studied our movements and took note of what the Chinese women might say to us. Usually we were surrounded by about twenty people, and these would come nearer and nearer. Sometimes they assumed threatening attitudes, and in such cases, we would decide to go on.

The previous day, two pretty young Chinese girls ran into us.

Achille said, 'Hey, let's talk to them for a bit and then take them up to our room.'

As he said this, however, we hadn't yet noticed that in the darkness many eyes were already fixed on us. I asked the two what their names were, and they told us, two nice Chinese girl's names, Ming Yi-Yi and Zhang Hua-He. They giggled and we indicated the route to the hotel entrance. They might well have come with us and even gone into the hotel with us, but before anything like this could happen, we found ourselves suddenly surrounded by a group of seven- or eight-year-olds who shouted at the girls accusingly. 'You should be ashamed of yourselves for going off with these two Long-Noses!'

'Da Bi-Zi' is an unpleasant title for foreigners – though there are worse. 'Long-Noses' – this is what these urchins called us. I went up to one of them, pointed to his small, flat nose and said with a smile, 'Ni hao, xiao bi-zi' ['Hello, you little short nose!'].

Uproarious laughter all round. Disturbed by the noise outside, the hotel porter appeared with a long face and asked me in English what was going on and what we intended.

'Nothing, actually,' said Achille angelically. 'We're cultivating friendship between peoples.'

'Then that's in order,' the porter said, and with a crude word or two he summarily shooed away the spying kids and the suddenly frightened young women.

'I feel just as though I were sixteen again in Strasbourg,' Achille remarked. 'Tried there, too, to find a girlfriend. It all comes back to me.'

I told Achille what had happened to me when I made my first awkward approaches to girls, and he, much amused, said that he had experienced very much the same. I went on to tell him, too, that foreigners were controlled in China wherever they went and whatever they did. This was officially justified as taking care of them so that they would not be exposed to danger of any kind.

Arrived back at our room, we found that we had received visitors in our absence. We discovered the administrative officer in charge of the doctors' groups, together with his interpreter for English. Either of these two were at liberty to enter our rooms at any time, whether bidden or not. Our rooms were not locked, and this I found to be an uncomfortable fact.

As we entered the room, both of them got up and came towards us in a dignified manner.

'Gentlemen,' they said, 'may we enter your room? We have one or two things to say to you.'

'You're already inside,' Achille said shortly. 'Fire away!'

In order to ease the tension between us, I opened a bottle of Kirschwasser (cherry brandy). 'Won't you take some?' I asked. At first they were not inclined to drink anything, but eventually were persuaded to indulge. There seemed to be something unpleasant in the air, something uncomfortable that they wanted to get off their chests.

'Well, now,' the elder of the two began, 'what were you doing outside?'

You see, I said to myself and threw Achille a dark look. *They've been keeping an eagle eye on us and there are going to be accusations.*

'Where have you been all evening,' the interpreter repeated, 'and why did you do that?'

I described rather clumsily the way we had taken into the town, but did not go into details as to why. The conversation limped on, and eventually it became clear what the two really wanted, and that was something totally removed from our suspicions. They merely used our diversion through the town as a means of introduction. It turned out that they wanted to give us some pocket money, which we would receive from the Chinese government in order to facilitate the purchase of odds and ends such as paper or writing materials or money for a haircut. The pocket money amounted to about 60 yuan or ren-min-bi, and this approximated to about what a Chinese worker earns in a month.

'It's for buying small items,' the administrator added.

We found this a remarkably kind gesture. Achille said to me quietly in German that we couldn't possibly accept this from these poor people.

'Many thanks,' he said, 'but we've brought our own money with us for such purposes.' I pointed out to him, however, that, according to Chinese custom, this would be considered impolite and result in loss of face by the Chinese.

'Do they want to buy our goodwill?' Achille asked. 'If we take their money, then we can no longer criticise them; we've been bought off, so to speak.'

'The most unpleasant thing about all this is their loss of face, 丢面子 Diu Mian-Zi, if we refuse their offer. On the other hand, we mustn't allow them to blackmail us. Somehow, we have to find a way out of this.'

'Then we'll accept,' Achille said loudly in French, 'but we'll award it straight away to the College of Chinese Medicine to use for special needs – for, say, the extension of the library perhaps, or for the purchase of certain teaching aids.'

We told our visitors of this and they were visibly impressed when I added that Mao's description of Chinese medicine as a 'Great Treasure' was also to come our way and so benefit us, too. The two men were very pleased at this and brightened up considerably after feeling that their offer had initially been turned down. 'We accept your kind offer,' I said, repeating my thanks, 'but I am quite sure that the college can well do with the money. It could even be that it needs the money more than we. After all, we have sufficient means to live in the West and don't really need the money, if you see what I mean.'

Having said that, I poured glasses of Kirschwasser all round, noting at the same time that our reasoning had pleased them greatly. Mr Lu said that if I wanted to stay in China after the course was over then I could do this for as long as I wanted.

'We are now good friends. And if you want to come to China again, whenever it suits you, you can. You will always be welcome.' I understood all this as typical Chinese small talk.

Achille in fact had once uttered the wish to come to China and work as a surgeon, in order to see for himself how surgery was practised here. For my part, I wanted to study Chinese herbal medicine and get to know prescriptions for treating internal diseases. However, I had already learned from Dr Kang that as far as this was concerned, there was no chance for foreigners to study these things. So a little goodwill at this moment wouldn't hurt anyone, I thought.

Two Female German Maoists

The lady at the German embassy in Beijing had given me the addresses of some Germans living in Shanghai, and these included two 'female Maoists'.

'These young women students appear to be quite lonely,' she intimated to me. 'As a doctor, do drop by and see how they are. I have noted from your *curriculum vitae* that you have been working in psychotherapy.' Apparently, my documents, which had been sent to the embassy from the German Ministry of Health, had been gone through thoroughly by this woman.

'They are often both ill,' she went on. 'They frequently seek contact with the embassy, although of course we're not here as soul comforters or even friends of our country people for that matter. For us, these persons are simply German citizens as we are. The Chinese party bosses are not so keen on ideological guests such as these, since they fear that once they realise that this country is not the paradise they had hoped for, they could lapse into disillusion, and after a time, they could go into the other direction and become haters of communist China.

Mao knew this syndrome. It was for this reason that he said in his small red bible: 'We are fighting as well against windbags and word-mongerers. The thinking of these so-called Leftists jumps over certain needful, objective developmental processes. Some of them hold on to their illusions as truth and others try to realise their ideals in the present, but too early for them to bear fruit. Such things lie in the future. At the present point in time they have cut themselves off from reality and in their actions prove themselves to be mere adventurers.'

The diplomat smiled her lonely smile. 'I'm here after all as the representative of the German Federal Republic and my boss says I'd better keep this kind of stuff to myself, but I like to do what the old Chinese used to do and keep the full truth hidden behind clever formulations. We diplomats live from the monies which flow from your pockets and those of other German taxpayers who are equally industrious. We know that, and you should know that we know. We are proud of your confidence in us, and wherever we can, we want to justify that trust.'

I stood there amazed at her openness.

'One of our unlucky Maoists could become prominent overnight, in the same way that you could become with your acupuncture. She would only need to write a book about everything she had experienced in Shanghai over the last three years. It would be a sensation. Here, it is really quite different to what you read about China in the West. As a result of such a book, she would suddenly become an interesting author and, of course, a taxpayer.

Well, there you are. One of them, by the way, has an eight-year-old daughter. She lives with her mother and attends a Chinese school. What does she learn there? A bit of bad Chinese, very poor English, and apart from that, a lot of stupid political claptrap. What's going to become of an otherwise nice kid?'

I found the telephone number of these two Maoists. They lived in a hotel near the college not far from where we were staying. When I rang them on the recommendation of the embassy, they promptly invited us to their place for a cup of afternoon coffee on the next day. They told me their address and the room number. We went on foot, the distance being not much more than a few hundred yards.

When we arrived at the reception desk of the so-called Friendship Hotel we were assured by the staff that there were no such people living there. The women we were looking for were apparently unknown to them. They pretended they had never heard of the names. This, of course, wasn't true; they merely wanted to prevent us from contacting them. Realising this, I asked whether I might ring them from reception. 'That's forbidden,' the surly receptionist told us. Nevertheless, I was not going to be fobbed off. 'Then please call this number for me,' I said to him, and shoved the note with the number on it under his nose. Now, whether he wanted to or not, he had no alternative but to dial the number. I could hear the same woman's voice that I had heard yesterday.

'You wait here,' the unfriendly Cerberus commanded. A moment later, a small, slim young woman stood before us. 'Please come upstairs; the coffee is ready,' she said.

We were cordially received when we arrived at the apartment. One of the women said that we could all go out to eat sometime, since that was possible. Achille and I agreed that we could indeed do that sometime. The small brunette who had fetched us from the hotel reception was pleasing to us both. The other was rather thin and a bit spinsterish. Yes, she had her eight-year-old daughter there as the diplomat had said. The child attended a Chinese boarding school and came home at weekends. The girl learned English there, said the mother, and had settled down in this socialist system very well, and had furthermore thrived on it, much better than in Germany, she said. Above all, the child had learned to accept things and manage difficulties well.

She was obliged to do a lot of physical gymnastics every day and as a result her body had developed well.

'Have you no men friends here?' Achille wanted to know. They shook their heads. 'Both of us were divorced in Germany. Anyway, Europe is a muck-hole. We don't need men in a socialist dispensation. Here, we enjoy the freedoms of a worker and farmer state.'

'What kind of freedoms are there, then?'

'Oh, there are plenty,' said the young woman, avoiding collision.

'And the disadvantages of the party, the police and the military?' Haubensack added drily by way of rounding things off. But the two women were at one in parrying his criticism.

The brunette then said, 'Mao was the first person in human history to give women the freedom they need. Here, we women are really free. There is a quotation by him which goes, "The time has come for women to be able to hold their heads high at last; the domination of the man is becoming weaker as the days go by."' She knew that phrase by heart.

'And Mao also said,' she went on proudly, '"Women shall be paid the same wage for the same work, since men and women are politically and economically equal. There are no differences any more between men and women." There's only one place in the world where this is really the case, and that's here in the People's Republic of China. And that's why I'm here and why Annegret and her little daughter, Gaby, are also here.'

There was a pause in which all this was digested.

'Shall I explain the difference between men and women?' Achille asked slyly.

'No, I'd rather not hear about it,' came the reply. This particular subject did not seem to interest either of them, but something else did.

'What's going on in European politics at the moment?' the women wanted to know. We told them.

The thinner of the two piped up excitedly, 'Last year we heard that the highest court judge in the land, a very devil of a man, who had hunted down our freedom fighters, Ulrike Meinhof and Andreas Baader, and locked them up, has at last been tracked down and killed by our folks.'

'Oh that. That was a cowardly murder,' Achille noted, but the two women ignored his remark.

'There's new hope for Germany because of this. We might even return if there were more of those rogues out of the way. Is there any chance of that happening?'

All this irritated Achille. He began now to draw parallels between the women with no sex appeal among the ranks of those living in communist China and the nuns living in medieval European cloisters. 'The nuns weren't allowed to have sex, apart from a few chosen candidates, with an abbot, say, or a bishop. And that's what it's like here; why don't you simply admit it?'

The women were much taken aback by this, and I could perceive a black cloud of ill feeling on the horizon, and tried to sweeten things a little, but it was no longer possible.

'What are you doing here in China anyway?' the skinny one asked crisply.

'We want to study acupuncture,' Haubensack said.

'And then take the thing to Europe and sell your knowledge at a price?' She looked at us bitterly.

'No,' I intervened, 'we want to serve the European people.'

The two communists nodded approvingly, while Achille for his part laughed contemptuously.

'That's more like it,' said the brunette. She added that she now had to go to the cinema, and left us sitting there. Her companion sat silently with a stony face. I felt it time to take our leave.

When we were back in the hotel room I received a lecture in the history of Alsace and Lorraine. In addition, I was at the same time receiving instruction in French. Achille corrected my grammatical errors and, in acknowledgement of my teaching him Chinese, widened my vocabulary with the addition of numerous words, many of which, I must admit, to use the phrase adopted by the *Oxford Concise Dictionary*, were 'not in polite use'.

Doctors and Religion

After dinner that evening, our group turned to the subject of religion. We had noted the various religions subscribed to by participants in the course. The Arabs among us had said, one and all, that they were Muslims. They believed in Allah, in his prophet, Mohammed, and in the Koran. Achille was of the opinion that all this was exactly the same bilge as that promulgated by Christianity, a state-stipulated belief in a Roman Catholic god and his church. This, he said, was the greatest criminal hindrance to humanity's further development. It was only a means of the Church inflicting itself on people to keep them malleable for its purposes, and in this way they returned to an infantile stage of development.

'What do you believe in, then?' asked the pretty young blonde, Adrienne.

'I believe in the power of enlightenment and in the continuing effects of the French Revolution, neither of which has yet had its day. And I believe in common sense. My favourite authors are Voltaire, Rousseau and Sartre.'

The young woman replied a little shyly that she had been brought up as a Protestant, but that religion was a lukewarm affair at home. The Dutch had accepted Protestantism out of political motives, whereas Belgium had remained in the lap of the Catholic Church. This had led to the separation of the country into its Flemish and Dutch components, although both regions spoke the same language. She herself had not seen the inside of a church since her confirmation, and whether she would marry in a church she did not know. If she were honest with herself, she would say that medicine was her religion, which she practised every day in order to help her patients. This is where she found her conviction and purpose in life.

The two men from Cameroon joined the conversation. Balu, the chieftain's son, said proudly that he was a Muslim, but he was contradicted in this by his companion. 'Nonsense, Balu, you're an animalist like all of us in Cameroon.' This was something unheard of in African social tradition. The truth was that Adnan had his place in that social tradition as a simple rural doctor, even if he was a medical director, but nevertheless he was well below the rank of a chieftain's son.

'Bullshit!' Balu countered, and kicked Adnan's shin several times quite hard, so that the latter cried out like a beaten dog.

'Merde! When I say I'm a Muslim then I'm a Muslim dammit! You can't tell me anything else!'

'It's not "animalist" but "animist",' Achille interjected. 'If you were an "animalist" you would pray to animals, but you're not that – or do you in fact pay honour to apes and rhinos?'

Adnan shook his head.

'As an animist, you believe in the activities of spirits, as indeed a lot of people do today in Africa. This would mean praying to the souls of these ghosts – that is, to their anima – and if we take that seriously it's not far removed from the feminine spirit of the Catholic Virgin Mary. For my part, I've never encountered the lady, but I revere women in general and for that reason Mary, too. Adnan has my support in this.'

Balu furiously dug his black heels into the sandals which were far too large for him. 'I don't care a damn about animist or animalist; I'm a Muslim and to the devil with the rest! Understand? I have a copy of the Koran at home. And now I want to go to bed.'

'Perhaps his old man, the chieftain, gets a rake-off from Saudi Arabia or Persia,' Achille whispered to me conspiratorially out of the corner of his mouth. Balu looked at him with hate.

'Whose bread I eat, his drum I beat!' ['Wes Brot ich ess, des Lied ich sing'] Achille intoned. 'It's an old Swiss mercenaries' saying. It was always so. And that's what it is – Hallelujah!'

The two Swiss joined the discussion and the surgeon from Lausanne, Claude Sifferelin, said that he was a good Catholic, but he was as inwardly convinced as his Dutch colleague that his 'church' was the operating theatre. There, he could speak daily with God, whenever he wanted. Sometimes, he added, God spoke to him directly while he was at work. For this reason, he loved his profession.

'Then you're really a genuine Swiss Protestant – we talk to our God personally and need no pontiff,' said Reto Armbruster, his colleague, a man stemming from an old-established scion of Basel physicians. One of his forefathers was Paracelsus' protégé, the illustrious Dr Armbruster, who was the editor of a book on herbs during the Renaissance and who, further, as a dubiously distinguished doctor, soothsayer and astrologer, made a name for himself at the Austrian court in Vienna before unobtrusively retiring to Switzerland.

'It's true of course that we Swiss put up the so-called Swiss Guard for the Pope's protection and that it is a relic of the days of Swiss mercenary activity, but at the same time we've had Paracelsus and Oecolampadius in Basel. Then there's Erasmus of Rotterdam who put the Pope on the spot and who even regulated Martin Luther and helped to initiate the Reformation. You could go on without further ado and without being shy about it be a reformed Swiss like me.'

'Oh, but let's have a bit of incense and the nice Catholic family ceremonies. What have we got in our dull world otherwise which we could attach our hearts to?' Sifferlin replied.

'Where is your heart, then, Claude?' Reto asked.

'That's just the tragedy,' Claude Sifferlin sighed. 'Everyone wants the incense and the family celebrations and yet all this is merely a superficial show, a kind of *panem et circenses*, as it was called when the Romans had somewhat come down in the world.'

'But that's not a suitable Latin quotation,' Achille carped. 'The Church has never fed anybody, it just puts up with a nefarious illusion. You should better say "*Mundus vult decipi, ergo decipiatur!* The world wants to be duped, therefore it should be duped." It's from the famous "Ship of Fools" published by an Alsatian scholar 1494 in Basel.'

'Well, what I really meant to say,' Reto said apologetically, 'is that we Swiss have much more in common with each other than our respective religions allow or would have us believe. So it's for this reason that we're really proud of our Swiss identity.'

'Is that still a religion at all?' the Frenchman Jean-Claude Giroudoux asked.

'And what about you, Ralf?' Adrienne asked in order to provoke me.

All of them went along with this question. 'Come on, you German acupuncturist, say something in defence of your religion, so that we all know where you stand and can put you in a pigeonhole.'

'You are nothing; your religion is everything,' said Achille disdainfully, insinuating the Nazi jargon of the '40s. He knew those years as a child, when Alsace and Lorraine were not only invaded by German troops but even belonged to what was then called 'Great Germany'.

How could I respond?

'You have something to hide from us?' they shouted.

I said nothing. All of them now fell into excited debate.

'You'll have to subscribe to something,' they demanded. 'If you have no religion at all, we won't be able to understand you. Otherwise you'll be like a passing cloud in the heavens, having no substance, a mere shadow. A nothing!'

'But of course if you are perhaps a member of the Chinese Communist Party you need not say anything . . .' Achille mocked. 'Then you would have a magnificent religion, the most beautiful that is to be had here in this proletarian paradise, and you could frankly boast of your membership.'

'I have a German passport,' I said simply.

This brought tumultuous laughter.

'See here, this is a German's passport!' Achille cried in feigned derision. 'These Germans travel everywhere, buy land for themselves, houses and other estate, and so spoil the pitch for others all over the world. In France, we have to pay more and more just because these bloody Germans still come over the border to us and then stay.'

At that moment I was put in mind of Lao-tse.

'I'm really a nothing. I'm an empty vessel. Every day, new information pours into my mind, which I then have to process. Above all, this is true here in China. Then, to this questionable "I" stemming from the Age of Enlightenment and the French Revolution, I have to take a stance. Should I begin to doubt whether there is an "I" at all? Perhaps in reality there isn't such a thing. What do you want from me? What I should do really is to tell you all about myself, my youth, both before and after the Nazis, my later career in Germany as a doctor. Perhaps then you would understand me. What use is it to me to be criticised by an Achille Haubensack? I'm an "I" like the rest of you, but I don't know yet what it means.'

'Mon Dieu!' Haubensack announced, 'now he's really gone round the bend!'

'Please let the others speak first,' I requested.

'Right, then. Let the Laotians have a word!' Haubensack commanded. He had suddenly become a small Napoleon.

'Oh, that's quite simple,' they said. 'There is the Tao; the Tao is our way, and the Tao is our time. Our old culture is there, because our life is there, just as the Buddha taught and it has been written long ago.'

'Come, now!' Achille boomed. 'You Laotians are communists anyway!'

'Yes,' they said gently. 'The communists are of course with us, but they don't disturb us one bit. Because in their hearts they, too, are Buddhists. The majority of Chinese, Vietnamese and Laotians are also Buddhists. The Buddha, as in ancient times, is still our saviour. That's how it will be in the future as well. The Buddha means happiness, life, success, understanding, and even science. He is all of those things, everything that you could desire. All you have to do is to let him into your life, dear colleagues and friends.'

'Oh, my God,' Achille said again with mock desperation, 'now that's a real convert's declaration! Do we all now have to become Buddhists?'

'The next Frenchman, please,' I said.

Giroudoux stood up, a trifle formal, a trifle affected, but for all that a kindly, charming man. He went on to give a perfect speech. That we had not expected.

'Dear friends, we've known each other now for only a few days, and find ourselves confronted with a new country and an entirely new type of person in its society, yet we doctors are a group with more or less the same interests. I'm pleased about that. You ask me about my religion. That's a ticklish question. Admittedly, I'm a French Catholic. That, however, is something different from a German Catholic or a Swiss Catholic. In Germany, the congregation receives its priest from the higher echelons of authority – that is to say, from the bishop, who, in turn, receives his position from the Vatican. As such, it is a congregation without a say in the matter. Its members have to accept the decision made for them from above, from Rome. That's how it has always been in Germany. In France, the parishioners elect their pastors democratically. As a consequence, they are seen as our personal priests, our own "brothers in Christ", so to speak, and people in whom we place our complete confidence. I like that, somehow. After all, someone must be responsible for the congregation's spiritual well-being. I can't do that as a doctor, not on my own as a doctor. I have six children, and my wife works with me in the practice. Together, we have a wonderful family life and I am happy to be a respected physician. The French Catholic Church supports me in this and gives me a feeling of security. So, that is why I'm a French Catholic.'

The other French colleague, Dr Albert Lagarde, the anaesthetist from Paris, said that he was in complete accord with the views of his colleague Giroudoux.

Now it was my turn again. But what should I say?

'Off you go, Ralf, it's your hour!' Achille shouted.

'Friends,' I said, in order to win a little time. 'Dear colleagues all! Whether you believe it or not, I have waited a long time for another chance at last to come to China. Why? You expect a few observations on my nature and the real nature of the human being – in other words, a few words about myself. But can I give you any such information?'

'Why is he going on like this?' Balu spoke up. 'We all want to get to bed now.'

Adnan, who had formerly been kicked by his companion into conformity, now pacified him by laying his hand on his arm. 'Let him talk. All day, we have to listen to the party's propaganda, perhaps we can hear something honest for a change. He is anxious to say something important and that's good for us all because it comes from the heart.'

I breathed in deeply.

'I was baptised and confirmed in the Protestant faith, but that doesn't mean a thing. Our vicars were a catastrophe. They were dishonest to a man and not far from being rogues. We knew that even as children as we watched their theatre performances in the church. And yet we had to allow ourselves to be confirmed by them. Without this formality we would not have been socially acceptable. My confirmation priest came regularly to my grandmother in order to pray with her because he well knew that she received care parcels from her daughter in America. After this little ceremony, he would beg for a couple of cigarettes and a tin of Nescafé, which he then received.'

I said all this in French, at the same time receiving black looks from Achille when I made bad grammatical mistakes.

'One of my ancestors was an evangelical vicar, a complete washout, a mangy dog who only brought misery to the family and finally drove them into bankruptcy. The beautiful old farmhouse owned by my great-grandparents had therefore to be sold.'

'Make it short!' Balu shouted.

'I'll be as short as I can. Four years ago, I left the Church, and from the taxes returned to me for this was I able to buy a fine Mercedes. I call the car "God's own car". I drive it around to the glory of the Almighty. There you have my religion. What do you want to call it? Call it what you will.'

Balu was suddenly quite awake and his mind was clear.

'A Mercedes for religion?' he yelled. He came over to me and threw his arms round me. He smelled horribly of garlic and now he suddenly spoke English.

'Ralf, my dear friend, please give me the address of your wonderful religion. I'll join your religious group immediately; they must be fantastic folks! I desperately want a Mercedes. This is the goal of my life. I love you, Ralf. Can I join your religion soon?'

'No, that's not possible, Balu,' I told him. 'You have first to be a member of this Church for a long time and you have to have paid a whole lot of money to the State and the Church. After this you can perhaps get the money back, and if the amount is enough for a car you can buy a Mercedes. What is paid in will then be paid back to you.'

'Then we'll have to change the laws,' Balu said threateningly.

'Have you got such things as laws in Africa?' Achille enquired.

'My father is a tribal chief; he can do these things. He can even force the stupid politicians to their knees and, when necessary, with weapons. He can summon up hundreds of thousands of fighters and he is always successful.'

He suddenly held his arms out wide. 'All of you. Come to Africa! Friends, we've got heaven on earth there.'

'If he weren't a Muslim I'd imagine him to be drunk,' Achille remarked.

'My father would do everything for you.'

'If you're Muslims, then there's no alcohol to be had at all, and that's nothing for me,' said Achille.

'My father determines what should be drunk and what not,' Balu cried. 'If my father allows it, then you can drink what you want, you can smoke and have many women, as much as you want.'

'And what about us ladies?' enquired the blonde Adrienne.

Balu looked at her with disdain, then noisily cleared his throat. 'You mean women?'

'No, we, us ladies', insisted Alice, the other Dutch physician, firmly.

Then Adnan put on his broadest smile. 'You will always be welcome, dear ladies, to our country Cameroon,' he remarked, trying to soften the controversial turn the conversation had taken.

'No!' snubbed Balu. 'Women are no real human beings, they are just things. I'm bloody amazed that your government has sent such sluts as you for studying in China at all.'

Adrienne shot up from her seat. 'That's an incredible affront!' she yelled. And Alice remarked harshly: 'From the mouth of a physician this sounds particularly rude!'

'For goodness' sake, let's get out of here,' said Achille quietly in my ear. 'Otherwise we'll find ourselves involved in a kind of civil war situation. Poisonous arrows have already been affixed and guns loaded.'

We all retreated to our rooms.

Conditions in Red China

We had just been strolling through a more remote part of the city along the Nanjing Road as part of a circular route. There were quite a few colourful corners on the way. Washing hung right across the road and people sat outside their houses. A toothless old woman pointed at us. The young girls sitting around her, about eight years old or so, covered up their faces immediately and Grandma feigned fear of us. It was probable that she had just said, 'Wai-Guo-Ren [people from foreign countries] are coming, these foreigners with long noses, and they'll eat you all up!' The children had stood up and wanted to run away, but as they noticed that we were friendly and did nothing to them, they began waving, then they laughed and jumped around. One young lad came quite close to us. He was interested in our cameras and when we made to go, he even gave us his hand.

There was one thing that disturbed me, and that was the total lack of privacy here. Achille Haubensack was always there, but that was just what the Chinese wanted. I could not wander around my own room; there was always someone in the vicinity. But this kind of thing is what is promoted in Maoist China. They call it the social life. Isolation is not encouraged. Our western idea of an 'I', an Ego is to vanish, and 'the masses' must take its place. One is not to live for oneself or promote the individual, to live behind closed doors and do things that shall be hidden from others. This is a fundamental principle behind the Chinese communist state's organisation. Mainland China's people have no idea of the price of this apparent social order. Their souls are offered up on the altar of the Communist Party. They are not individuals as we understand that concept in our European tradition, and they can never achieve that which we recognise as a personality.

Even more distressing than the destruction of the 'I' or, say, the lack of possibilities for its development is, equally, the repression of the 'Id', the libidinous drive from which every healthy human being lives and develops. It is probably the greatest crime of all that Chairman Mao cultivated the personal cult of a demigod to its highest degree, to the point of being an ever-present, all-powerful, all-controlling 'Super-Ego' so that his compatriots, or better, his subjects were brutally robbed of every opportunity for personal growth. For the European, a life such as this on the mainland is no longer of any value. It is total slavery, much more effective than anything comparable, such as what we usually view as the slavery that once took place in western societies.

One afternoon, for example, I had given lunch a miss because I wanted to do some exercises. This was something I could not do in the normal way of things, since I was never alone. Exercises did me a lot of good. As for the meals, we got the same kind of swill every day which was in general far too fatty. So it was not much loss to skip a meal. I was going through the cycle of exercises when two interpreters suddenly appeared to check what I was doing on my own. I happened to be standing on my head when they arrived. They had never seen anything like that before and looked rather foolish as they hurriedly departed. I said nothing to them and just remained comfortable standing on my head.

There is something I have to report concerning the course. We had a lot of medical questions that we wanted to ask of our teachers. We were usually told that our questions would be attended to after the lesson, since the teachers were too tired to enter into discussion whilst teaching. This, we were told, could wait until the evening. But then when evening came, none of our questions was answered, and certainly nothing could be spontaneously discussed. There was a constant need to remind our tutors and to insist on answers to our enquiries. Put in other words, what we were confronted with was a programme that was reeled off to us; it was not a genuine academic course in which one was an integral part of a university syllabus. That was not what was offered.

In the evening, I was in the so-called Friendship Store. The service in these places was execrable. The reason for the ubiquitous lethargy one found in them was that there was no motivation for those who worked there. The saleswomen saw not the slightest profit from their work. No one was interested in any kind of service to sell anything or even to advise and assist. I found myself waiting a long time until a tired, buxom lass stirred herself sufficiently to sell me a nail brush, and she evidently did so against her feeling. Upstairs in the textile department, the same atmosphere prevailed. For the salespeople there I was just thin air. They were not willing to show me the different kinds of shirts they had in stock and that I would have liked to purchase. They talked loudly to one another and treated me as though I were an annoying interruption of their so-called working time which, for them, was simply a matter of hanging around, talking about this and that, smoking and drinking tea. No people's economy can come to anything like this.

Any kind of question that concerned the articles on display earned at best a shrug of the shoulders. What was most clear was that there was absolutely no interest in the customer. When the sales personnel suggested something to buy and there was a question about it, the ware was immediately put back into its box and the customer was left to his own devices. Purchasing anything at all with money in hand made the customer feel like an enemy of the state. This, too, must be one of Mao's infamous doctrines. I found exactly the same slovenliness in the stationery department. I just could not see any plain white paper, only lined paper. Not even a simple white writing pad could I find.

Today, one of the professors, the one who related the history of Chinese medicine to us earlier, asked me in the academy whether anything was known of the Yin-Yang theory in Europe, and whether for me this was a completely new area of knowledge. I told him that I had known about this for years and used the concept daily in my practice of acupuncture at home. He just did not believe me. I tried to make it clear to him that there were certain similarities between Chinese traditional medicine and ancient western medicine. The passage-of-time concept, for example, the bipolarity of fire and water, the change from day to night, and the influence of the climate and the seasons also played a similarly important role in the theories of the early Greek physicians such as Empedocles, Heraclitus and Hippocrates, as well as for the early European philosophers. However, it was obvious that this professor didn't understand a word of what I was telling him. Again and again he asked me about the names of the people I had cited and wrote them down. The cultural history of the ancient Occident is for Chinese doctors in particular totally unknown territory. All of them are of the opinion that, as Chinese, they are the only custodians and masters of a practice of medicine that is unique in the world, a fact that I personally have always doubted.

But perhaps our lack of understanding of each other had something to do with our interpreters, one of whom was a man we referred to as 'Kipper' or 'Fishface', who was no great mind. This man was thin and undernourished. He wore nickel-framed spectacles with goggle-like thick lenses, which, unfortunately, made him look like a fish on legs, and it was for this reason that we gave him his nickname.

This 'Kipper' used to practise the right spoken tones in Chinese with me on the bus in the morning so that I could improve my pronunciation of Chinese. He had a strong Shanghai accent, however, and so could not give me the best of Mandarin intonation as a Beijing speaker could do. I had mentioned this on occasion and he admitted it, at the same time telling me by way of an apology that every region in China has its own pronunciation. This difference is so exaggerated that the folks in the north of the country cannot understand those in the south. The characters in writing, however, are everywhere the same, and so, because verbal communication is, if at all possible, very difficult, one has to write things down or write them in the air or on a partner's palm to be understood.

I noticed that this interpreter had a special dictionary for translators with him. This book contained a large section for medical terms and I asked him where one could buy such a book but he shook his head. 'That's not possible. This book is only for Chinese, not for foreigners'. That was the case everywhere, especially concerning books dealing with medicine, and medical terms were withheld from foreigners. The same was true for a book that came to hand recently, a French–Chinese medical dictionary. Our interpreters used it every day, but we were not allowed even to look into it. Fishface, who had apparently taken a liking to me, had promised to secure an English dictionary for me to look at one evening. 'But no one must know about it,' he whispered to me. Whether such a thing would be possible at all was another matter, since everyone knew everything about the other. There were no secrets here.

When anybody came to the hotel on a visit, like the two German Sinologists today, their names were carefully registered at reception, so that no one had unofficial contact with us foreigners. This was expressly in our own security interests, Achille was told as he started to protest. Such visitors could be burglars, for example, who could steal all that we have, or someone might intend physical harm or even endanger our health. It seemed that our hosts were much concerned about our personal welfare. This was one of the reasons, we were told, why we were transported by bus each day from the hotel to the hospital. So that nothing of the kind mentioned above would happen, we were not even allowed to buy a cycle, as I had originally intended to do, since we could conceivably have an accident with the thing.

Our journey to the clinic proceeded very slowly. The hospital was only about two or three miles away, but the trip took thirty minutes. This was an opportunity to talk to each other, read or simply peer out of the window to watch what was going on in the city. After the visit to the clinic, we could relax in the bus and I was glad to be able to read Chinese texts aloud and find Fishface or another interpreter to assist me in correct pronunciation.

Homesickness for Europe

I had brought a few tapes from home to play European music and could do this on my Dictaphone. This provided shades of home for us. Haubensack and I drank the appallingly sweet Chinese red wine to it and indulged in our imaginations about what we could do to relieve our bleak situation.

Achille said that among the twelve million inhabitants of Shanghai there were six million women, and among these at least two-and-a-half million women of our age and disposition. 'They would have nothing against meeting us privately and, despite this fact, we sit here sadly and meditate upon Chinese medicine.'

The music I had brought along put us into a slightly better mood. Compared with European music in general and with Bach's Brandenburg Concertos and Mozart's operas and symphonies, which we were currently listening to, Chinese music was quite primitive, and to our western ears, insistently boring.

Achille went on to complain. 'Above all, this sexual repression. It's like being in a concentration camp. Perhaps you know, Ralf, that there were women even in Nazi concentration camps for the needs of the men. We've not even got such a thing as that here. As a result we're much worse off than the prisoners in a camp. We find ourselves here in a nation which has three thousand years of history behind it and there is nothing to do except become slowly depressed!'

'The European music offered here is dreadful, too,' I added.

Once I attended a concert in Shanghai together with one of the interpreters. We went to a symphony performance where, as a first piece, there was a Chinese composition, a violin concerto with a Chinese soloist. In terms of the European rules of harmony it was a miserable failure. There was one musical construction error after another, parallel fifths and octaves for example, and the whole was very clumsily orchestrated. Although the violinist possessed a speedy technique to some extent, there were sections that were frankly amateurish, and it was pretty clear that the player had received no formal violin lessons in the classical sense of the word. Then came Tchaikovsky based entirely on a Russian performance example. There followed a tremendous thumping and banging, a row which had better never been attempted in the first place. The brass section especially gave rise to false sounds among the trombones and French horns and there were moments when wrong notes were just randomly and mindlessly thrown into the swell of the concert.

This made me ask the interpreter whether the orchestra had rehearsed the piece at all.

'Oh yes,' he said. 'The wrong notes are produced by members of our political party, who here have to work in every unit. And that includes orchestras as well of course. These folks are mere amateurs. They just play by ear because they can't read a note of music. They don't need to either as the party regards it as revisionist and bourgeois to do everything as perfectly as it is done in the West. Nevertheless, these cadres are all very fond of music and so the party has appointed them to perform in our orchestras.'

I told Achille of this cacophony. All he could do was shake his head.

'What can we do about it? Here we're like prisoners, and we'll just have to get on with it.'

A bit later, Achille said, 'But we must change things, even if it's only for those medical colleagues who come after us and who want to pursue a similar course. We're the first pioneers of European medicine who have come to the People's Republic in order to study acupuncture, and for that reason we are responsible for the coming generation of students. After all, we're concerned about our health and the well-being of our colleagues. It has been proved that a four-month sexual abstinence is not particularly good for one. Later in life that kind of thing can lead to prostate cancer or something similar. It remains to be seen whether the Chinese government is willing to accept the costs in such a case. They're just indulging in an infamous experiment, that's all.

'Theoretically,' he continued, 'we're being informed about the harmony of Yin and Yang. Yang is the man and Yin the woman. What's happening here is that there must be a harmony between the European Yang and the Chinese Yin and that is missing. This is absolutely against physiological rules and cannot be at all in line with Chinese medicine. As European doctors, we must protest and so start a counter-revolution. We're not very demanding in our situation.'

In the morning, while in the bathroom, Achille always sang the Communist Internationale. He sang this with all he'd got and his pleasant tenor voice was only interrupted by occasional hefty gasps as he stood under the shower. He liked to sing the Chinese national anthem, 'Dong Fan Hong', too. 'The East is Red,' it goes. After that, he would come out fresh and grinning to join me in the parlour, where he would further enlarge on the hideous inadequacies of Chinese medicine as practised in the People's Republic in general and on those of the idiot Chinese who practise such medicine in particular. After this we would go down to breakfast.

III

Getting Used to Chinese Clinics

A Chinese clinic can be recognised from afar by the penetrating stink of urine it exudes. This stench emanates from the toilet 'facilities', which are mere holes in the ground in every corridor and every ward. Often enough, this smell is joined by that of fresh faeces. What in European clinics is the odour of disinfection, formalin or chloroform is here the pong of Shao-Bian, as the Chinese say – in a word, pee. This wasn't any different in the Lung-Hua Hospital, the university clinic for Chinese medicine in Shanghai where we studied.

Early one morning we were shown one or two moxa techniques. A Chinese teacher burned up a moxa cone on a slice of ginger. Achille fell into ecstasy. He suggested that the Africans among us should now do a native dance around the patients' beds. This, he said, would induce an even better placebo effect. Adnan Kirinin was immediately ready to oblige. He felt the rhythms already in his legs and his massive body began to sway gently to and fro; his eyes rolled up and down and his head turned from left to right. This earned him black looks from Balu and the Chinese teachers, as well as from the interpreters.

Achille suggested to the Chinese professors that the huge African could bring his tom-tom from the hotel tomorrow morning and then, adorned with a feather headdress, lead the moxibustion ritual through its phases. The method would work much better, he averred. However, the interpreters were not ready to translate his proposal, since there were 'too many unknown words' in his proposition, words which could not be found in their respective dictionaries.

We laughed until our sides ached. I have the suspicion that the name 'Kirinin' was originally a derivative of the German word 'klein' (small), endowed upon the family in colonial times. That would be an interesting antithesis not only of the man's huge size, but also of his pitch-black skin. After the unhappy affair with the proposed totem dance, which he would have been very glad to have obliged us wth, he now dismissed my suggestion about the origin of his name with huge arm movements, thick, pursed lips and rolling eyes, saying, 'No, no, Kirinin is a genuine African name! A lot of families have the same name in our country.' Then he laughed until he could hardly stand. His body shook with pleasure and he hammered on his huge, broad chest with his fists, which indeed produced a sound not unlike that of an African drum. In all this, he roared and struck poses, shouting 'Je suis le Gorille!'

Alice, our Dutch colleague, collapsed during the burning of the moxa. Suddenly she lay on the floor with her arms outstretched and her face green. We got her on her feet again after dosing her with a glass of Lao-Shan mineral water. As she came to, she told us that she never entered a smoking compartment on the railway, because the smoke always made her ill. 'Is there no non-smoking area in the clinic?' she asked desperately.

However, our teacher shook his head. 'It's always the same with Chen-chiu,' he said, 'that is, with genuine Chinese acupuncture. Moxibustion belongs inseparably with it. As Europeans, you don't know that. You just go ahead with the needle application.'

The Chinese physicians are smokers practically without exception. They smoke for the very simple reason that Mao Tse-tung was a chain smoker. While applying acupuncture in the clinic, they just hold the burning cigarette in their left hand, inhale the smoke and then go on placing the needle into the patient. No patient would ever think of objecting to this custom, and even if he did, he would receive short shrift from his clinician.

The Dutchwoman protested that everywhere stank from morning till night. There was a ubiquitous stink in every therapy room. She doubted whether she would be able to stand this until the end of the course. Indeed, we asked ourselves what was the most penetrating – the stench of moxibustion or the smell of urine.

Chinese Organs of Thought

Today, there was an excited encounter between us and our professors when one of them announced that the liver, the kidneys and the heart contributed greatly to intellectual ability and to the ability to think. Our western colleagues, led by Achille Haubensack, protested hotly in the ensuing discussion that they in no way thought with their livers and kidneys, but, like other Europeans, with their brains. The professors let us know via their respective interpreters that we were not here to discuss Chinese medicine, but to listen and so learn about the subject. Chinese university instruction just consists of copying and repeating what the professors offer to their students. It was just not done to argue with one's professor, dispute his claims and debate the toss. We in turn argued that we could not learn without doing so, but the Chinese could not understand this at all. They informed us that if this were the case then we had the worst of manners, and they told us this in so many words, which is actually very un-Chinese. They were clearly extremely annoyed.

Achille, however, was very upset and said via his interpreter, 'Now, please translate what I say and exactly what I say. What your colleagues have just said is totally opposed to classical anatomy and modern physiology. I admit that sometimes men think with their willy, but not since the origin of Man has anybody, at any time, thought with his liver or with his kidneys!'

The interpreters again refused to render this into Chinese. Then, silently, the professors and all the other Chinese went out of the room, and we were left to ourselves. The other lessons for the morning were cancelled.

Yesterday we saw acupuncture in practice for the first time. We were appalled by the primitive conditions and the prevalence of filth everywhere in Lung-Hua Hospital. I had been there three years before on a fourteen-day information course and it was exactly the same then as today: unclean and run-down. The walls had dirty patches which had not been re-painted or obliterated, and here and there the red brickwork showed through. Moreover, the little plastering that remained was now peeling off in places. In addition to all this, the doors were greasy and hung crookedly on their hinges. All the windows were open to the sky, and as a consequence, a fresh wind blew in from the Huang-Pu River.

Patients lay ten or twelve to a room, men as well as women, young and old, all of them in one ward. Some of them sat crouched on chairs. None had really undressed for examination and only small areas of flesh were visible. In this, they were typically prudish Chinese, prudishness having had a long history in China. In earlier centuries this led to the need to diagnose patients by the state of their tongues or the condition of their pulse, since no one wanted to undress in front of the doctor.

In the annals of the imperial court we read that the doctors there were never allowed to actually see the sick empress. Three strands of cotton were tied to her wrist and then led through a keyhole to the physician sitting outside. He then had the task of making the correct diagnosis of the lady's complaint from what he could feel in his hand. Because of this, he was obliged to develop para-psychological and para-diagnostic abilities in order to survive. For God help him if his diagnosis was wrong or his medicine failed to help. The doctors of prominent people were quickly dispatched should they make mistakes. The profession of a doctor was not held in much esteem in those days.

The relics of this kind of prudishness is still to be seen in Shanghai. This is in stark contrast to patients in the West who, without shyness, will take off their clothes and lie on the examination couch without demur, sometimes quite naked should this be necessary.

Hygiene is also something that is a lax matter here. It suffices to dab the skin with a swab doused in alcohol, and often even this simple procedure is overlooked. We asked whether the needles are sterilised before use, to which we received no answer. The doctors treating the case simply use their bare hands, taking the needle and administering it, withdrawing and applying it to the next patient without cleaning it. One operator, a somewhat older doctor, puts the needles into his mouth after application. He holds them there in a bundle all together between his stumpy, tobacco-brown teeth before he treats another patient or before putting them all together in a bowl. The needles are not then later cleaned or sterilised, but just used again on other patients.

The burning of the moxa herb is a special attraction. In Europe and elsewhere it is referred to by its Latin name, *Artemisia vulgaris*, a plant which is as widespread in China as it is in the West. All the techniques using this herb were shown to us while we were there. Using this technique, a moxa cone is placed on the skin or a grain of moxa is then burned there, producing a wound on the skin which later heals leaving a scar. If applied to the chest, it is supposed to be very good against asthma. In Europe it is not possible to perform this because of the injury that ensues. A woman came into the room with stomach pain as the result of drinking cold liquids. A slice of ginger was laid on her abdomen and then a moxa cone was placed upon this and the whole was ignited. As a result there was cloud of stifling smoke as it roasted and hissed. The air was so thick with it that our Dutch colleague again fainted and had to be carried out into the fresh air by two nurses.

We now came to a critical phase in our course of study. We had left our initial enthusiasm for China and its medicine behind us and found ourselves looking a bit deeper into things. We noticed the dirty fingernails of the doctors, which remained filthy all day long, and we criticised what for us was a miserable interpreter team. Often things were so badly translated that even I with my meagre knowledge of the language could correct them. I felt the need to control what they said. 'That's not correct,' I would say. 'The professor said something quite different from what you interpreted!'

At this, the majority of the interpreters merely shrugged their shoulders. They were just too lazy to do their job conscientiously. They were simply looking forward to their next meal. There was nothing more important to them than this, Chi Fan. They were pretty indifferent to everything else.

The Importing of Earplugs is Forbidden

Each night we suffered from the incredible row from outside that issued from the harbour, the river and the road below the hotel. Because of it, I lay awake for hours every night and could not get to sleep. Sometimes I took a book to the bathroom and read there, as I didn't want to wake Achille, who enjoyed a sound, deep sleep. As a result, I was tired during the day. The majority of us would return to Europe today rather than tomorrow.

Yesterday there was notification of a parcel from Germany waiting for me to pick up. I was obliged, it said, to fetch it personally. It was probably my earplugs which had arrived and which would ensure me a little more peace at night. The postal official opened the parcel in front of me and pulled out a small box, and said: 'These must under no circumstances be sent to China; I will have to return them.'

'Why?'

He pointed to the name of the manufacturer. 'There is the name of a pharmaceutical producer – in other words, that means these are medicaments. For this we need special governmental permission that we haven't got in this case. The import is therefore forbidden.'

I ask the man to open the box so that he could see for himself what was inside and how harmless the things were. He did so.

'There you are, you see, just cotton wool and wax.'

'On the packet it says "Chemical/Pharmaceutical Goods", and that's what counts, not what is inside.'

'Hey, wait a minute!' I said. 'I'm in service here as a doctor and a better judge of what this is than you are. I need these as ear protection against the terrible noise at night.'

'You might be a doctor in Europe, but you are not a Chinese doctor,' said this arrogant civil servant.

I was furious. 'If I don't receive these earplugs, I shall leave tomorrow.'

'Please yourself,' said the post office official.

I was greatly annoyed by this and still upset by the time the afternoon lecture began. I told Professor Xiong of the incident and he promised to help me. He wrote a prescription for the earplugs and sealed it with the university's stamp. A few days later, Fishface handed the things over to me in the hotel. Grinning all over his face, he said, 'There we are, now; aren't we Chinese the friendliest of people? We do everything for your benefit and for your health.'

At last, I can sleep a little better.

We Adapt Ourselves

Yesterday, Achille and I bought so-called Mao jackets and caps in the Friendship Store. We arrived dressed like this for the evening meal, much to the great amusement of our colleagues.

The Chinese, too, were impressed. They said that now we had almost become real Chinese. Not one of them noticed that we were only having them on. Perhaps they didn't want to know. It was very difficult to get behind their faces which, as we've said before, had to be safeguarded at all times. Afterwards, we went into the town in this new attire and it was astonishing that now the Chinese pedestrians took no notice of us, whereas the weeks before when we went walking in our European clothes they had all looked at us without exception. Both men and women had called after us or had laughed at us or made rude remarks to the tune of 'Long-Nose!' or something equally impolite. Children and others had even pulled us by the sleeve to see whether we were actually real people of flesh and blood, or ghosts perhaps (in Chinese: Gui), or men from Mars, automatons and robots.

Three years before, an old woman in Shang-Sha had screamed in panic and made the strangest, inarticulate noises as she discovered me in a shop. At that time I wore a thick, dark brown beard, something no Chinese has, and, on top of that, I have bright blue eyes, which is another odd thing for a Chinese. She kept crying out, 'A ghost, a ghost!'

No one in the shop who tried to console her in her panic could convince her that I was not a demon. On my previous visit I happened to be in the city of Hang-Zhou on the top floor of a large store buying stationery when I discovered that all the other Chinese customers had followed me upstairs in order to take a peek at me. Finally, several hundred had assembled to register my every movement and satisfy their curiosity, astounded that I could make my needs known to the Chinese assistant in their own language. As a result of there being so many people on the top floor, there was a real danger of the rundown building falling into the road, and for this reason the manager authorised the removal of all those other customers, who had to leave the building, and I was left to make my purchases entirely alone. However, it was a pretty uncomfortable as well as boring business to be left there alone in this huge store to wander around and be silently gawked at by sales personnel, so that I soon made for the street again. This would not have happened in Mao clothing, as at least from the back I would have looked like the rest of Chinese humanity.

We had the suspicion that all our mail was opened and read. The ambassador in Beijing had presaged this, and one or two remarks on the part of our interpreters confirmed our feelings. We now knew that the interpreters, young people of both sexes, were familiar with our personal data in the fullest detail. They, in short, knew everything about us and we knew virtually nothing about them. Weeks ago, I had written a letter of complaint to the ambassador about the unbearable noise from the street at night. The authorities had certainly read the letter, since, lately, there had been a marked decrease in the noise intensity at night. For perhaps three or four nights it was noticeably quieter, but now that was all over. Despite the earplugs, I still managed only to sleep a little and could hardly keep my eyes open during the day.

Chinese 'Meridians' and a Childbirth

We were now studying the so-called meridians, and I tried to explain to the interpreters that the European term is a misleading one. They just showed me their dictionaries. In them, for the ideographs 'Jing-Mai' and 'Jing-Luo', the word 'meridian' appeared. I told them that this was wrong and showed them the old traditional character for this term by painting it for them and analysing it. They were quite unfamiliar with the ancient Chinese concept because they had learned a new, sino-communist attenuated form of writing. I invited them to come up to my room, where I had a book by Leon Wieger in which the old, more complex traditional characters could be seen together with their explanations.

One of them in fact did come along, but either he could not or would not understand my objections. He resorted again and again to his own dictionary. For him, everything was in this book, and when the party publishes such a book, then it cannot possibly be wrong. With that, he wished me 'Good night' and left the room.

The woman doctor who was talking to us today about the courses of the meridians over the skin, the Jing-Luo, used a black felt-tip pen to show their routes. She had spent some time in Africa, and at that moment she was dealing with the heart 'meridian'. With our black colleagues she used a piece of white chalk in order to better demonstrate the necessary contrast on the skin. It looked much better somehow than the black lines on our white skins. Again, the interpreters told us that they could not translate this observation.

'It's a damn pity I can't speak Chinese,' said Achille. 'I'd show these nincompoops which way the wind blows!'

Our black friends had to put up with a lot of teasing, but took it all in very good part. With the exeption of Balu, they were thoroughly decent people – above all, our rotund Adnan. Nevertheless, they had some difficulty with the two ladies in our company. These were young, modern self-confident doctors and therefore for our Africans, who didn't think much of women anyway, something of a puzzle and an embarrassment. Wherever they could, they avoided speaking to them as they didn't know quite what to say and so felt uncomfortable.

The Chinese do not tolerate any mixing with blacks. If, for example, a Chinese girl becomes pregnant by a black student, say, the party decrees that she abort immediately in order, according to the Chinese view of things, to avoid producing what they imagine would be a terrible monster. In the case of white mixed-race children there is more tolerance, but authorities are inclined to recommend abortion as well. The quota of abortions to births is 1 to 1, which means that for every fifty births in the People's Republic, there are also fifty abortions. I learned this on a recent visit to the gynaecological department of the Hua-Dong Hospital to which I was invited, since I was the only colleague among us who had had training in midwifery and, as a medical practitioner, I had delivered many hundreds of women.

I was allowed to be present during a childbirth. The woman had been prepared with four acupuncture needles to reduce pain. Two of these were in the San-Yin-Jiao on the inner part of the lower leg and the other two were located on the back of the hand, the He-Gu. The midwife twisted all four points every few minutes to stimulate the effect. The birth was easy and quick. The newly born baby had the typical dark blue Mongolian patches on its bottom. The umbilical cord was cut and the child began to cry. The mother was very happy, she laughed and was delighted with her child. The only child she would be allowed to have, it was laid on her belly. If she were to be pregnant once, twice, three or four times again she would be obliged to abort on every occasion. This I learned from the midwives, and it is a heavy burden for the Chinese who are, and always have been, lovers of large families. For them, this Communist Party law is a terrible test as it drives young women to request that their fallopian tubes be resected immediately after their first child is born.

Chinese Security and the First of May

One of the things that struck me the previous night while walking through the city was the feeling of security that there was here, even in the darkest corners and alleys of Shanghai. We now always wore our 'Mao' uniforms and nobody took the slightest notice of us. In the evening, the people here walked slowly and thoughtfully along the streets. They gave the impression by their attitude that nothing could happen to you; your personal safety was assured.

In western countries this is not so. You have to look out for yourself on the street so as not to be knocked down, or so that no one seizes your purse, and you have to take care that nothing is thoughtlessly forgotten or left lying around. Here, anything lost or forgotten is with certainty delivered to its owner in the most remote corner of the land, and especially if that owner happens to be a foreigner. Three years ago, a group of visitors, including myself and comprising pharmaceutical chemists, doctors and university people, was here. One of our company threw a frayed toothbrush into the rubbish bin in his room on leaving the hotel. The train for Canton had to wait for half an hour in the station because the chambermaid had found this brush in the waste-paper basket and rung the railway station. Later, on the platform she happily shoved the tired instrument over to its owner personally through the carriage window. He was completely flabbergasted and told her that he didn't want it; it was on its last legs and really quite useless. Regardless of this objection, he had to take the utensil and was unable to get rid of it in fact until we reached Hong Kong, the last port of call on our journey.

Apparently, the security system works very well in this country, so that even in Shanghai, once a city of ill repute, there is little theft and few crimes. Theft, for example, is severely punished. Once we saw a number of men standing on a truck, their heads close shaved and with placards hanging from their necks on which was written in Chinese 'I am a thief' and 'I was caught stealing'. These men were surrounded by an indignant crowd who not only pointed their fingers at them, but actually spat at them in contempt. Frequently enough, the Chinese authorities apply the death penalty in petty offences, especially for political divergence.

This gives everyone a certain security within the political system, but at what price! It is at the cost of personal freedom, which is something the people here entirely lack. Certainly, there are other negative factors to this system, which we as privileged foreigners would never encounter.

Today was the First of May, Labour Day as it is called in the United States. Nobody was at work; instead, everyone was out on the streets. All of us were invited to a festival where there was a circus, clowns, jugglers, dressage, music and singing conducted in Shanghai's stadium, which could accommodate about twenty thousand people. The place was full to the last seat. The spectators had brought their own food with them so that there was a smell of fish, meat and vegetables, rice and fruit. People talked loudly during the performances. These filled three hours without an interval and finally the programme became an intolerable bore as one feature followed the other and every number was similar to the last, and they were sometimes repeated *ad nauseam* – at least from our European point of view. They were all more or less the same, involving praise for Chairman Mao and for the Revolution.

Foreigners in Shanghai and a New Bicycle

The other evening, I received a visit from a German student learning Chinese here who told me that the contact between Chinese and foreigners is deliberately thwarted. Every Chinese can reckon on encountering difficulties when he has anything to do with a foreigner. He also confirmed that the post office controls letters, not only those of foreigners living in the country, but also those of the Chinese themselves. It then often happens that letters are wrongly placed back in envelopes, although the post control officers continuously deny this even when they are caught. The worst feature of all, though, is the oppressive, omnipresent and all-powerful bureaucracy invading every area of life, the pedantic exactitude practised in the smallest administrative matters and in insignificant detail, and the mutual prying, sneaking and spying which even infests family life. Here, it is less pronounced than in Beijing, he said, but in his opinion the Chinese are thoroughly insincere, so that they can whitewash their lies with ease. They expect the same from foreigners. As always, the most important thing of all is to keep face. Rather a lie, even a big lie, than risk confrontation with facts.

We came across people who apparently did not benefit at all from the new order of society. One of these was the ragged fag-end collector whom we met one night some time ago in the Nanjing Road, and another was the drunken clochard of whom we have already spoken, people who because of their unreliability or because of their political past were not entitled to a pension and who were not allowed to go abroad, even when they would do better there. This student felt that China was anything but a paradise. He had spent eighteen months in the country so far.

In my letter of complaint sent to my ambassador in Beijing I also mentioned that I would like to buy a cycle, but that this was denied me, since responsibility could not be taken for my safety in Shanghai's traffic. Yesterday, our group leader, Mr Lu, surprised me by saying that in the Nanjing Road there was a very good cycle shop, and that the bicycles there were not at all too expensive. If I wished, I could buy myself one, but only there and nowhere else. Accordingly, I went over to this shop and bought myself a very heavy but nevertheless stable black, shiny Chinese cycle. I noticed that it had no back-pedal brake of the kind common in Germany, but only two hand brakes, one for the front wheel and the other for the back. I had to get used to this. I paid for it in cash and it cost about 80 Deutschmarks at the time or roughly 40 euros today – in Chinese currency, 78 yuan or ren-min-bi.

In the shop, I was asked where I worked in Shanghai and to which unit I belonged. I told them I worked at the Shanghai Academy of Chinese Medicine as a European Chen-chiu doctor.

'Very good. When you work for us you get a cycle, but not as a usual foreign tourist.'

The next question was whether I could ride a bike at all. 'Yes,' I said, 'I can.'

'We'll have to test you,' the salesman said.

I replied that this was all right with me. Air was pumped into the tyres and every part of the cycle was examined. Then someone carried it downstairs from the first floor of the building to the street below. All the personnel in the shop came out to look. I swung my legs over the crossbar and set off to do a short trip and then back to the shop, where I was greeted with a round of applause mixed with laughter. Yes, this Wai-Guo-Ren, this 'Long-Nose', could cycle almost as well as a Shanghai rider.

Then I set off with a feeling of the greatest safety and joined the tidal wave of Shanghai cyclists flowing with many thousands of others on their way along the streets of the city. Of them it is said that they almost never have an accident, because everyone takes appropriate care. A cycle is a treasured possession and not cheap for a Chinese. The average worker in China receives a monthly wage of about 60 yuan. As I was wearing my Mao jacket, no one took the slightest notice of me and consequently I felt myself to be a Chinese among other Chinese. I started out first in the direction of the port and from there headed towards the suburbs of the town, which I had never visited and to which we were never allowed to go. Here, the way people live is appalling. In many of the houses one can look straight into the bedrooms. The windows are open for all to see and now and again there are people lying in the beds. Some people live in two-storey houses, which here are something of a luxury, and usually the bedrooms are on the upper floor. The houses stand in filth. Their inhabitants sit outside to eat, probably because it is cooler there, and in any case it is too dirty inside. They eat their simple white rice from bowls with chopsticks. Children play around them. Everywhere there is lumber and trash, a chaos of rubbish and abandon; nothing is tidy or well-cared for.

On the way there I recalled a Chinese character that I wanted to teach Achille. It was that of a pig under the roof, 家, and meant family, home, the place where one belongs. It was an appropriate illustration for these conditions. As I rode along I caught the attention of the people around me; people nudged each other and pointed at me. Little girls laughed and waved to me. Here, in the Shanghai suburbs, no one had seen anything like this before. A wooden bridge came into view. It probably spanned an arm of the Huang-Pu River. I crossed it and made for the harbour. Looking down, I could see people in sampans, little boats, appearing very similar to those in the bay of Hong Kong. I felt fit. The exercise had done me good after weeks of mostly sitting around, and the next night I slept soundly.

More Chinese Characters

Once back at the hotel, I related my experiences on two wheels to Achille.

'What do you think the Chinese character for "home" or "family" is?' I asked him.

'Well, I imagine that it would include a woman and child,' he replied, and took up a pen and paper.

'That's how it is perhaps in Europe, but in China it is something different. The pictograph is a little more complicated than the previous ones. Let's first of all draw a roof,' I suggested.

He drew a pointed roof after the manner of building in Europe.

'Chinese roofs look a little different,' I said. 'Have you ever seen one? They have a kind of ridge, too, but the slope of the roof is not as great as it is in our latitudes. By the way, we've already drawn a roof of sorts – heaven – so if you like, we can begin with that.'

Achille drew a horizontal line 一.

'Now place a point at the top and that's the highest point of the roof.'

He did so 亠.

'Now put guttering all round so that the rain can run off.'

This was achieved by placing a tiny vertical line on the left and right: 宀.

'That's the Chinese roof under which much can take place, as with us. You can't write the whole character for "family" yet, so I'll show you.'

I put the pig, 豕, under it.

'The Chinese character for "family" is a pig under the roof: 家, pronounced Jia.'

'Is a Chinese home a pigsty then?'

'In a way, you can say that.'

'Is that why they won't let us look into their private houses?'

'We'll have to assume that.'

'Now put a woman under the roof. What could that mean?'

'Housewife.'

'Not quite, but something akin to that. It means "peace", "an", 安, which, in ancient China, was something that came about when a woman was in the house. When you place "yu", 玉, jade, the emperor's jewel, under the roof, then that means a treasure. Write that now, it's pronounced Bao.'

Achille wrote 宝.

'If you draw an "eight" under the roof, then that means "cave", a dwelling below ground or a hole in the earth.'

'How do you write an "eight"?' Achille asked.

'Ah yes, let's write "eight", Ba, 八. Then we want to write the rest of the numbers. "Four", for example, is "si" and written like this: 四. As you can see, it's a square with two vertical strokes in it because this number can be divided by two.

Achille drew the number 'four', 四.

'Then a "five", 五, "wu". This is to represent the five elements, or better still, the five seasons. It comprises four corners and a middle, like this. Originally it was drawn as a cross, so draw the cross first.'

He did so: 乂.

This cross was drawn between heaven and earth, the Yin and Yang, in order to represent the five elements. We know this from our lessons we've had at the academy.'

Achille then drew heaven and earth, 二, as the upper and lower borders for the cross of the five elements, 乂.

'Out of this developed the modern wu, 五, for the number five. You can see from this that there is a piece of Chinese world cosmography in it. The next divisible number after four is six, and you can see this by the two strokes of the number eight, 八, below an upper line: 六, liu.'

'Number seven consists of two strokes, 七, and has a simple explanation, I went on. 'It is pronounced "ch'i", 七, and sounds as if you were about to sneeze. Incidentally, it is used as a radical in the Ch'en or chen, 齔, sign and indicates the appearance of the second teeth in human children around the seventh year of life. In this way, every Chinese character tells us a little story.'

Achille drew 七, the number 'seven'.

'The eight, too, consists of two strokes, which signify division, since the eight can be divided four times by two. This letter, 八, Ba, is the lucky number for good fortune as luck comes up whenever things are divided and shared among people. The number nine, 九, "Jiu", is simply a figure denoting “nine”. It arises from three times three; this means that Yang, 三, can be multiplied by itself and has a particularly strong quality. All the classics in Chinese literature consist of 81 chapters (nine × nine) because this produces a particularly strong Yang effect.’

Achille drew the number nine, 九.

‘Number ten, “Shi”, 十, is the number of complete perfection. It is represented as a cross which points in all four directions of the compass, and at the same time, it symbolises “middle” or “centre”. As you know, China is the “Middle Kingdom”.’

Achille drew this, too.

‘Beginning with these quite simple principles, the rest of Chinese numbering is very easy. You can place the basic numerals next to one another.

Eleven is ten and one: 十一, Shi-yi.

Twelve is ten and two: 十二, Shi-er.

Twenty is twice ten: 二十, Er-shi.

Twenty-one is twice ten plus one: 二十一, Er-shi-yi.

Twenty-two is twice ten plus two: 二十二, Er-shi-er.

Thirty is three times ten: 三十, San-shi.

One hundred is that which shines brightly under the roof: 百, Bai. One hundred can as well be written as 一 百, Yi-bai.

Three hundred is three times hundred: 三百, San-bai.

One thousand is: 千, Qian (or Yi-qian, 一 千).

Three thousand is: 三千, San-qian.

Three thousand six hundred and fifty-nine is three times a thousand plus six times hundred, plus five times ten plus nine: 三千六百五十九, San-qian Liu-bai Wu-shi-jiu.’

‘That’s much easier than our Arabic numeral system in fact,’ Achille said when we went down to the bar for the odd glass of beer.

A Talk with a Colleague and it is still the First of May

Yesterday evening I sat with Dr Kang, one of our teachers, in a hotel room. We had been acquainted with each other for three years. He was active in research, whatever that might mean here. I asked him what his particular branch was, but he sidestepped my question. It was clear that his area of ‘research’ was ‘secret’.

‘Library’ was all he was willing to divulge. I wanted to know more, however. And the work he was at present working on? What exactly was he writing about?

He hesitated for a moment. Then it appeared that he was currently writing an article to do with the Nei-Guan, which was a certain acupuncture structure near the wrist on the inside of the lower arm. In general he seemed to agree with me that Chinese medicine must first prove itself to be scientific. He had studied both, some basic western medicine and Chinese medicine, but for only a three-year period. He came from Shanghai and had completed his studies in medicine some ten years previously. We agreed to meet more often, because I had a few specific questions to put to him and he seemed generally interested in an exchange of opinion. This was certainly a special exemption, because I had no 'paper' permitting me to meet him privately.

Yesterday, on the First of May, there was a great show of fireworks which lasted for two hours and was very expensive, but that is something which the party is only too glad to present to the people. The most beautiful garlands of falling sparks and flower patterns could be seen and rockets shot into the sky above Shanghai without pausing. Millions of bulbs illuminated the city for a couple of nights, and this, too, must have been enormously expensive, but this big spectacle was all part and parcel of the party's desire to impress the people. In the Europe of the past, emperors and kings launched similar spectacles by erecting architecturally monumental buildings. In 1936, Hitler, the German dictator, staged a colossal Olympiad in order to demonstrate his powerful political influence to the world. The same was true of the Catholic Church in Europe, for which no pomp and splendour was too much if it were the means to convince the faithful of its God-given power. The same took place here this evening, only that in this case the Chinese people's god was alive only three years ago and his name was Mao Tse-tung. Those who have unlimited power can allow themselves such display. Such a thing would be impossible for a western democratic state, although it must be added that the Germans privately squander about 40 million euros annually on fireworks at New Year's Eve.

Yesterday we celebrated the First of May and no one studied or worked on this day. A boat trip was organised for us. Once at the harbour, we went aboard a ferry which took us down the Huang Pu as far as the open sea – the East China Sea. We had hardly travelled along the river for ten minutes when we were told that we were not to use our cameras any more. This was in the interests of preserving the military security of the Chinese state. We had to pack away our cameras under the sharp eyes of our watchmen.

Then we sailed along the river. On either side there was nothing of the slightest interest to be seen. No ship passed or overtook us. We came to a provisional landing stage, and there we could see old submarines and a rusty gunboat built in the style of the 1920s, old iron which in Europe would have long been melted down. It looked very much as if these old ships had been bought up cheaply after the Second World War. This port, which was once the focal point of trade with the world, was more or less defunct. I caught sight of four ships, a Norwegian vessel, a Dutch ship, two boats flying the flag of Panama, and that's all. The heyday of Shanghai as a port was over.

The air was cool. The closer we got to the open sea, the more the waves splashed on the deck, and everybody was suffering and feeling queasy. So we all went below to hide from the cold and the dampness on deck, those classic disturbing elements responsible for illness in Chinese medicine. There we all squatted miserably under the galley and drank mineral water. Although we were allowed to smoke here, we merely sat and dosed.

In the afternoon, I went off again on my bike with a Swiss colleague and the blonde Adrienne to a well-known teahouse situated in a small park. In the meantime, by the way, two other colleagues had received permission to purchase a bicycle. In Shanghai a lot is made possible if one perseveres long enough to get what one wants. Before long, we had a swarm of Chinese folk behind us anxious to get a closer look at us. They watched what we did with our bikes, how we got on and off, our movements and how we locked our cycles and what we actually did before going into the teahouse. The Dutchwoman had straw-coloured hair, and this assured her the attention of the unlookers. Small children pointed their fingers at us; some were frightened and hid behind their mothers' skirts. Hardly had we entered the park precincts when a spy appeared to track us down and carefully observe what we did. He remained behind us at every step, and followed us wherever we went. Above all, he was anxious to prevent us from photographing anything. But he was not able to hinder me from taking photos of alleyways with a wide-angle lens. When I approached a table at which two elders were playing cards, he roughly intervened by shoving himself in front of the camera. He didn't allow me to push him aside either, and stood there like a concrete block, never once looking at me or saying a single word. When I again raised my camera for a shot, he sprang out of the shadows with ape-like alacrity and placed himself between me and my subject. I thought to myself at that moment that this man was specifically trained for this kind of thing, since no untrained individual would be capable of doing these things with such skill. In addition to his gymnastics, he had availed himself of the help of a throng of young boys. If he was not quick enough to do the job of thwarting my camera shots, then the kids were there at once, holding their hands over the camera lens and looking at me cheekily. The whole manoeuvre was not aggressive, but was thoroughly aimed at checking any attempt to take photos and frustrating us in our activities.

It was clear that those watching over us felt irritated that we were allowed to wander about in this area. For us, it was by far the prettiest and most Chinese of all the places we had seen. There was no doubt about the fact either that if photos were taken here, they would not reflect the fame of China if they ever came into the hands of a western newspaper publisher. In the West, we have the impression that everything in China is kept backward. People exert themselves at least superficially, but the government is always at the forefront of action. However, it cannot be said that even one objective – even the most trivial – has been achieved. This can be directly applied to things medical. One works with what is to hand, and this is often done very skilfully, but having said that, everything is well below European standards. There is an admirable lack of prejudice in the application of acupuncture and Chinese medicine, but it cannot for a moment be said that this is a modern form of healing that will one day overtake modern western medical knowledge and practice. I have put forward this viewpoint in Europe, and it is interesting to note that it was confirmed here in practice, by which I mean it was confirmed by reality, and more clearly than at any other time.

Medical Brainwashing, Bad Food and Ageing

We had a sneaking feeling that the medical theories served up to us in Shanghai were a kind of brainwashing. The diagnoses that were presented to us, such as dizziness, hernia, acute appendicitis, spermatorrhoea (an unusual illness affecting Chinese men who suffer from the involuntary loss of semen), were definitely not scientifically corroborated, but were just empirical assumptions that did not accord with our western medical concepts. We were confronted on a daily basis with blasts of such undigested assumptions. The result was that we were hardly aware of the fact that we were gradually becoming immune to these senseless statements and unthinkingly or mechanically taking them for granted. We had to watch out that we did not lose our critical medical mind, otherwise we would find ourselves accepting any kind of statement as the truth without question.

Every day, the Chinese practised their Tai-Ji-Quan exercises on the street in groups in front of the hotel and began with these at five in the morning. One of the Maoist women we visited came over from her hotel and also took part, and I came across her later in the foyer of the hotel on the ground floor. She maintained that through these exercises one acquired a sort of general feeling of common identity with the universe, of being one with everything, and that when these exercises were practised, one was no longer an individual, but became one with all the others. I was amazed to hear her say this because she had appeared to be rather an activist leftist when Achille and I talked to her and her mind-mate at their hotel. This experience, she said, produced a very harmonious atmosphere. To exercise alone is something less well known in China. The individual is not as encapsulated here as in western countries. It probably was the feeling of being completely dissolved in a mass of people that fascinated that ideologically thwarted woman. Could this perhaps be a so far undiscovered feature of the subconscious background of militant communists? Do they really want to dismiss our European idea of the Thinking Ego, the 'Ego cogito' of Descartes?

As a result of the fatty food and the lack of exercise here to which we were more or less condemned, most of us had put on weight and so felt pretty uncomfortable. The food was not particularly rich in content, and as a consequence, we were always hungry again after a few hours. This in turn led to our visiting the so-called Friendship Store in order to buy extra bread and food of some sort. Cafés of the kind known all over Europe where one can take afternoon tea or coffee together with a piece of cake are unknown here. The Chinese drink tea with their food; the Persian folks, the Syrians and we Europeans drink beer, which changes the digestive properties of the food we imbibe. In fact, Chinese food is not amenable to alcohol. Many Chinese cannot stomach beer at all, not to mention wine or schnapps.

In passing, it might be mentioned that the Persians and Syrians in our group looked much older than they actually were. The fat Syrian cardiologist, for example, was only fifty, but looked seventy. The other Syrian was forty-four, but looked as though he was in his mid-fifties, perhaps because of his habitual careworn expression. We decided to call him 'Mr Misery', because he looked so downcast. The professor for anaesthesia from Damascus was only forty-seven, but looked as though he was in his mid-sixties. Apparently, people age at different rates according to the climatic zone in which they live. We western Europeans lie somewhere in the middle of the two extremes. The Chinese, for their part, are very difficult to assess when it comes to judging their age. Even when they are well over forty, they can appear to be about twenty, and one can only judge their age by their grey hair. However, on the other hand, most Chinese people dye their hair as soon as the first grey hairs show up. Only one or two women doctors here, for example, actually appeared grey-haired in public.

Every day in the evening in our hotel room I studied new Chinese pictographs with Achille.

'Back to the roof, 宀, and the number "eight", 八, then,' I said. 'From the combination of these we come to a character which is important in Chen-chiu, acupuncture. Draw this now.'

Achille painted the eight under the roof: 穴.

'This character is transcribed "hsüeh" in the English Wade–Giles rendering and written "xue" in Chinese Pinyin transscription. It depicts a cave – that is, an underground dwelling with a path which leads deep into the interior. Our teachers describe it as a "point", but this is wrong. A point is named "Dian", 灬, in Chinese. You can see already for yourself what oddly muddled things we're told here. You see, there are no acupuncture "points" as such at all!'

'Have we come all this way to learn that?'

'We have to be careful that these people don't tell us more hair-raising nonsense!'

Achille shook his head in disbelief. 'What idiots do they think we are? As a surgeon I can't say I agree with what they're telling us.'

'But you are still learning some Chinese characters. An important one is the sun, and that you can draw straight away.'

Achille drew a circle, ○.

'Now place a point in the middle,' I urged. 'That's the old sign for the sun, "Ri", ⊙. Later, the dot was lengthened to a line simply for convenience and speed in writing.'

Achille drew Ri, 日, 'the sun'.

'It also means "a day" or "daily". Ri Bao, 日报, is the daily newspaper in China.'

'And the moon?' He drew a half moon, ☽.

'Very good,' I said. 'It is simplified to give an open double arc with two lines in it, like this: 月. This is spoken as "Yue". At this point you have to be careful. The character looks exactly like the abbreviation for "meat" or "flesh", Rou, and mustn't be confused with it. This shortened form, 月, is one of several signs concerning structures, organs and the bodily parts of the human being. First of all, we'll paint the character for "flesh" or "meat", Rou, 肉. It is supposed to be the representation of a dried piece of meat. Then we'll draw the character of the moon, 月, Yue. This character for "moon" is used for the word "month" and everything which has to do with this, even including a woman's monthly period. If we now put both "sun" and "moon" together, this will give us a new character – namely, the character Ming, 明, which means brightness, clarity or a radiant beam of light.'

Achille drew the character Ming, 明.

'The famous "Ming Dynasty" was named according to this concept. If you want to buy a Ming vase, as you say you want to, then you will need this sign to make yourself understood. From the "sun" 日 character we derive the term Bai, 白, which means bright or white; if we then put a line above the sun, we have "heaven". This is white, clear and bright like the sky when the sun rises. If you put the two together, we have Ming-Bai, 明白, which means "to understand". It has a similar meaning to that which we refer to as "enlightenment", or carrying light into the darkness.

'I'd like to do just that,' Achille said.

'It means that kind of enlightenment in which you believe and which is not yet at an end in Europe as you say. Inasmuch as it is this, it is your leading star.'

'I would not have understood it without this character. Did the Chinese experience such a thing as the Enlightenment in our European sense?'

'Of course. But this is kept secret in today's communist China, because free thinking is not allowed. This lack of freedom to think is bound up with all the hocus-pocus we're bombarded with here.'

'Am I to understand, then, that modern China is a dark country compared with earlier Chinese dynasties or with the classical epochs of European development?'

'Above all, compared with the cultural epochs of the Occident, yes, one could certainly say that.'

Now Achille had learned another eighteen characters, making thirty-three altogether.

A Very Private Encounter

I had the opportunity again to speak in private with Dr Kang. At first we talked about the meridians. 'The meridians,' he said, 'were lines drawn after it had been ascertained that certain constellations of points had a common effect on certain organs and bodily structures.'

'First the points were there,' he explained, 'then came the connections or "meridian lines" joining them. Later in ancient China, and as a result of anatomical studies, it was discovered that these lines had their parallels inside the body and that these ran in courses similar to those found on the skin. The Chinese anatomists discovered that the blood vessels were hollow enough for bamboo twigs to be placed in them. The nerves and sinews ran parallel with the blood vessels and with groups of muscles. From this they concluded that the lines on the body surface represented vessels and nerves along which blood and Qi flowed.'

'In other words,' I said, 'the description we find in the book *Huang-Di Nei-Jing* is a later explanation of the "meridians"?'

Kang laughed and showed his long yellow teeth. 'That's possible,' he replied. 'I wasn't there at the time when the *Nei-Jing* was written. But there were forerunners to the version we know today, stemming from the Tang Dynasty (AD 500–700), and it's pretty certain that the old text was often modified.'

I said that the idea of the meridians being canals as such is not scientifically tenable and that it is a pre-scientific conception, which was far from being even a hypothesis, to which he replied: 'We assume today that the meridians are closely connected with the peripheral nerves as well as with the blood vessels.'

'An objectification, a real proof, has not yet been demonstrated by you in China, and the Korean Kim Bong-Han's claims in the '60s that he had proved the meridians and points anatomically were quite clearly disproved. But Kim maintained that he had substantiated the existence of the acupuncture points and also "shown" the existence of the meridians. Kim committed suicide, as is well known here and elsewhere in the Far East. He did this because he had made statements in his publications that were false, and so he lost face.'

Kang agreed.

I took some paper and a felt-tip pen and drew the classic symbol for 'meridian', Jing, 經, and explained to him what Dr Wieger had to say about this.

'The first part, the radical, is a tangle of silk, 糸. The horizontal line on the right is a surface under which a small stream flows. This represents the surface, 一, of the human organism under which the blood vessels, 巛, flow below. This upper horizontal stroke, 一, is the skin of the human organism. There follow three small water courses, 水 (abbreviated as 氵), below this surface which can be researched by touching and feeling. The latter is denoted by the character Ting, 工, which is now somewhat abbreviated. According to this, the "meridians" could then well be the blood vessels of the human body just below the surface of the skin, which can indeed be felt and where the pulse can be detected. Apart from this, also of interest is the fact that the lines of longitude on the globe – that is to say, the vertical lines on the globe, our western meridians – are altogether different in Chinese – namely, Zi-Wu-Xian, 予年线, sometimes also referred to as Jing-Xian, 經线. In the case of the last two characters, the first, although it is written the same as Jing-Mai, 經脉, its meaning is altogether different here as the second character refers to a line and not to blood vessels.

'How come that you understand so much about our old characters?' Kang asked.

'I've been interested in them for years,' I replied.

Dr Kang was quiet.

Then he said, 'Here, we only know the Mao Tse-tung form of writing, the simplified versions of the written characters.'

'Then you can no longer read the original texts?'

'Oh yes, we have had a lecture on the ancient medical language at college.'

'Did you attend these lectures?'

'Not regularly. I never had enough time. I always had too many patients, and on top of this were the necessary party meetings and Revolutionary Committee gatherings. In Europe you are in a much better position; you have more time to study than we do here. I would like one day to go to Europe, indeed I would! Many of our Chinese doctors would like to do that as well!'

His pale yellow cheeks had assumed a dark red colour and his black eyes were protruding. He looked very excited.

'Did you know that there were early anatomical studies in ancient China?' I asked.

For a while Kang remained silent. Then he said, 'No.'

'It's mentioned in the book *Huang-Di Nei-Jing Ling-Shu*.'

'Where in there?' Kang asked.

'In chapter 12, entitled Jing-Shui, 經水, the imperial physician Qi Bo, 歧伯, mentions anatomical studies of the structures of the human organism to the emperor, Huang Di, 黄帝. He says: "After someone has died, his body can be anatomically dissected for medical investigation."'

Kang shook his head and said: 'But this had no influence on the development of acupuncture in China!'

'I assume that what are called "meridians" today probably to a certain extent were the result of such anatomical investigations,' was my reply.

'Sorry, I'm not allowed to talk about such things with you,' he answered stiffly. I understood. The Communist Party did not allow him to touch upon certain subjects with me. So we had to find another topic for our conversation.

We went on to talk about the Five Elements and their application in acupuncture. He said: 'The party with its revolutionary new orientation in today's China has declared the Five Elements as unscientific. The teaching of Ying-Yang, however, is still valid and is also regarded as scientific. We refer to it as "the dialectic of Chinese medicine". It is the same as that propounded by Marx, Engels and Lenin.'

'Well, dialectic thinking actually comes from Hegel, who took it over from Plato, the Greek philosopher.'

'The Chinese communists don't go as far back as that,' Kang commented. 'That's too European, too much bourgeois metaphysics in it.'

'How far back do you go, then?' I asked.

'Only as far as Mao Tse-tung,' came the sobering reply. 'That's enough.'

I said: 'In the West the mistaken ideas of Chinese "meridians" and "points" of acupuncture are still widespread; they are taught in acupuncture circles and even by certain professional "needle societies".'

'Some of our old Chinese doctors – for instance, Doctor Ou-Yang in the clinic – adhere to such antiquated ideas as well. They would therefore need a refresher course,' Kang said.

'There are "needle gurus" in Europe, for example, who consider just these things as the wonderful "secrets" of Chinese medicine.'

' "Gurus", what are they? The word comes from India, doesn't it? We have nothing like them here in modern China.'

Oh yes, you have, I thought to myself. *You've still got Mao Tse-tung, and he's your super guru!*

'In Europe, and as a result of the general lack of orientation, we are quite susceptible to such tricksters,' I said.

'That's amazing in view of the fact that you have such high eduction and so many good universities.'

'The problem is that we have such a huge array of the most diverse and contradictory ideas and viewpoints that no one knows what the right view is and what not. It is a prime time for seducers of all kinds.'

Now Kang quoted something from the Mao bible: 'Mao Tse-tung once said, "Idealism and metaphysics are the simplest things in the world because everyone can talk a lot of nonsense about them, and without offering a shred of proof taken from objective reality. Dialectic materialism, on the other hand, needs effort to understand. It can only be founded on objective findings. Without this orientation to reality, we fall back into idealism and metaphysics." '

Kang had been strictly schooled as a member of the Communist Party.

He went on to say, 'The teaching of the Five Elements has been carefully investigated by us in the People's Republic. As a result, we have had to dismiss it as something falling short of reality. That's how it is with other ancient theories associated with Chinese medicine as well. That which is accepted has been crystallised from what stands the test of scientific proof, either under objective examination and investigation or from the point of view of its practical application.'

'The last is the main thing,' I said, and Kang agreed. 'When is acupuncture dangerous?' I asked him.

'It's dangerous when it's in the hands of amateurs – in the hands, that is, of those who are not properly trained and not doctors,' he replied. Again, he showed his long yellow teeth, but now his face had assumed the appearance of a rigid mask. Suddenly he seemed to have changed his mind about what he was permitted to disclose to me. 'People like that are unfamiliar with human anatomy,' he continued.

'Anatomy?' I was sceptical after his earlier remarks.

'Yes, anatomy!' he called out, and at the same time he looked quite embarrassed, since I had obviously caught his dissimulation. In any case, he didn't want to lose face.

'Our ancient Chinese physicians were pretty well acquainted with anatomy, you know!' he insisted.

'That's what I have assumed.'

'Well, think, for example, of the "Copper Man", the Tong-Ren, from the year 1026. His creator, Wang Wei-yi, was a genius in the matter of anatomical description of the structures of the human body. Western anatomy came much later, in the sixteenth or seventeenth centuries, if I'm properly informed.

'That's quite right.'

'At one time, one of the reasons why mistakes in treatment arose was because patients did not undress themselves fully,' Kang continued. 'The doctor was obliged to stick his needles through clothes and so had to more or less guess where to place them. You've seen for yourself at the clinic how bashful people are, and how reluctant they are to remove articles of clothing, especially the elderly.'

I then asked Dr Kang what kind of preconception or idea the traditional Chinese doctor has when he thinks of his patients.

'As far as this is concerned, the Yin and Yang functions play a great role. The older doctors, as I said, also proceed from the concept of the Five Elements, which is something we cannot entirely eradicate at once. For example, Ou-Yang, the older doctor at Hua-Dong Hospital where you practise, is one such. In this case, the doctor is familiar with the basic structures of the human body, in addition to the Shen, Qi, the blood and the body's juices. Further to this knowledge, he is also acquainted with the teaching on the storage and hollow organs, the Zang-Fu. All of them are very experienced in the use of the so-called transport lines, the Jing-Mai or Jing-Luo, which, as you explained today, we are no longer at liberty to call "meridians", because the old characters, as you said, describe something else.

Our traditional doctors are particularly aware of the role the kidneys play in producing Qi, the so-called innate or primordial Qi, and of the important living elixir, Jing, which the human being brings into the world from his parents when he is born. He knows well that this inborn essence, which in Chinese is called Xian-Tian-Zhi Jing, the essence before birth, must be constantly replenished by nourishment. In this, the stomach and spleen play an important role. For that reason, the human being must eat well and regularly. It's from this that the Chinese derive their love of food – something you have noticed every day in the clinic and at the hotel.'

Kang had spoken quicker and quicker in a low voice, probably because he had become quite nervous.

He described this understanding of what is inborn and what is acquired as the very essence of the Chinese art of healing, and also as that which basically differentiates it from western medicine. After an hour's conversation he looked tired and exhausted. Had he perhaps involuntarily stepped beyond the permitted limits? As we were certainly bugged and our encounter was secretly taped, his party colleagues would later on tell him.

Achille had just returned from shopping in the city at the moment Dr Kang was taking his leave, so at this juncture I felt it fitting to start right away with our Chinese characters for the body structures that Kang had just mentioned.

After our evening meal, we dropped into the bar for a beer.

A Visit to the Factory

Our group visited a pharmaceutical manufacturer. Here, western medicaments were made: cortisone, Butazolidin, Reserpin and Rauwolfia preparations, a few antibiotics and pain-killing drugs. The means of manufacture were similar to those used in the West, except that the machines were rickety and completely old-fashioned. One could assume that they stemmed from the Ming Dynasty! However, preparations were also made from Chinese traditional herbal prescriptions, and one of these was an anti-cancer recipe which was supposed to be effective against malignant growths in the stomach and intestinal tract. I asked Dr Kang whether this had been clinically tested. A little embarrassed, he laughed and said that this drug was mainly there to give the patient hope. Cancer patients in China were almost always informed of the dangers associated with this disease and, whenever possible, operated on early enough. One could not leave them to their fate without modern medical assistance.

'So it's just a placebo?' I concluded. But Kang did not know what a 'placebo' was. Actually it means 'I will please' when literally translated, and it is embedded in the western doctrine of the separation of body and mind. Thus, it concerns all those therapies that place suggestive effect in the foreground over and above the processes of an actual physical illness. Nevertheless – and I knew this from my researches for my dissertation while working in a psychosomatic clinic –placebos are responsible for 30% to 40% of all cures. Dr Kang found this very interesting.

'That goes very well with the concepts of Chinese medicine,' he said. 'Only we never sever the body from the soul here,' he added, 'and that would in any case be against traditional Chinese medicine and Mao's teaching. It would be a kind of metaphysics if we were to do so, and therefore it is forbidden. And in fact the two are just one in reality. Without Shen' – he wrote the character 神 on a piece of paper – 'which enters into a human being at birth, in addition to the inherited material Jing, 精, of the embryo, which is the primordial substance, the inborn Xian-Tien Zhi Jing (innate essence), there would be no human being capable of living. This Shen is later in life stored in the heart, Xin, 心. A Chinese thinks, feels and decides with his Shen and with his innate kidney power from which the will is derived. This is why there was such a discussion during class the other day about the meaning of the various bodily organs for thinking. You western medical men, well trained that you are, just can't grasp this.'

'Not yet,' I said and laughed. He laughed, too, but it was the usual snigger of the embarrassed Chinese.

I had received a letter from the German embassy in Beijing which included a question from a patient in Pakistan who had been a paraplegic for years and who would like to be treated here in Shanghai. I was obviously considered as a source of information and as a general intermediary. I had already received a large packet from the female diplomat in Beijing that contained a medical report for a Canadian patient who wanted to have her gallstones treated by traditional Chinese medical methods and not by the usual operational procedure. However, I was not allowed to practise medicine here in the People's Republic, although this would not be the case for Hong Kong. Perhaps there would be a possibility for her there. In any case, I would have to deal with this whole thing at a later date.

IV

First Patients in the Clinic

I had taken up my work at the Hua-Dong Hospital, which lay in the west of the city about two kilometres from the academy. Dr Kang had been officially announced as one of my personal teachers, and I was glad of this because we got along well together. On the first day we were greeted early in the morning by the Revolutionary Committee in the courtyard of the hospital. All the doctors at the clinic had been called together and now stood to attention during the course of the whole ceremony. No one moved a feature. It was as if they all wore masks.

We went up the broad steps to the first floor of the hospital. Everyone received a doctor's white coat, so that the Chinese could see that we were real physicians. At the top in the outpatients' department, we seated ourselves around a large desk. Tea was distributed from large Thermos flasks and we relaxed for a moment or two. Again, our interpreter, Xiao Gu, a small, pale woman with high cheekbones, the one who had been so irritated at Da Shan Hotel by Achille's Chinese characters a few days before, now began to hold another political speech.

She launched a violent tirade against the 'Gang of Four' (to whom Mao's wife belonged) because they had not been able to meet the requirements of the party line. While she spoke, Miss Gu's face had assumed a whitish complexion and the circular openings of her pupils got dilated, which could clearly be observed even though the irises of her eyes were naturally dark brown. The whole body of that little woman trembled with utmost scorn. These political affairs seemed to influence the whole life of each party member. I asked myself whether it was perhaps a family squabble that had led to a political battle involving the whole country. Everyone knew that Mao was a notorious skirt chaser and as such not a particularly pleasant man to be married to, but everything is allowed among the party elite. In Hong Kong some years ago I had learned from my journalist friend, Johnny Li, working then as one of the editors of the *South China Morning Post*, that Mao was not always an exemplary husband. Rumours of many a girlfriend and bed companion in the company of the great chairman would often make the rounds in secret among the women comrades of the hour. Whether these affairs led eventually to the condemnation of Mao's wife was debatable.

Hua-Dong Hospital was built at the time of the Japanese occupation. It has the reputation of being an especially good hospital, one favoured by high-ranking party members who enjoy a special right to be treated there. Today, modern western medicine is combined with Chinese medical treatment in caring for patients. At least, this is what is claimed. There are departments for internal medicine, gynaecology and midwifery, surgery, orthopaedics, neurology, ENT, eye diseases and acupuncture, as well as a children's department. Altogether, there are 270 beds for in-patient treatment, and in the outpatients' department, roughly 2,000 consultations take place per day. About 600 people are employed here, and of these, 110 are doctors, 140 are nurses and sisters, 50 are pharmaceutical chemists and 50 are physiotherapists. Over 100 clinical doctors of the hospital are obliged to work in the country as a kind of mild punishment for not conforming to the party programme in some way, such as, for example, being politically insufficiently informed or ideologically unstable. No one goes from here into the barren countryside unless he is forced to do so.

We had six patients in all on this, the first day of our practice. We were only allowed to look on, though – we were not permitted to treat them. The majority in our group were absolute beginners in the art of administering acupuncture. For this reason, we had a lot of theory to imbibe beforehand, and this was always imparted in the morning lessons at the college.

When patients came in, they laid their health card with its photo on the table. The first was a man suffering from migraine. I had been treating this condition for about the last five years in my practice at home. By profession, the man was a technician at a research institute. His symptoms were typical: pain always on the left side of the head, after much reading generally worse, bad in spring and often accompanied by sleeplessness. His tongue was thicker at the edges and also of a bluish-red colour. His pulse was tense. Kang wanted to tell us that it was a so-called meridian illness, which is the official term here, and I was reminded of our recent discussion. According to my opinion, this was a typical liver disturbance. The proof was the state of the tongue and the tense pulse. I whispered this to Kang in Chinese.

'This is not a meridian illness but a liver disease.'

He looked at me, obviously a little annoyed at this, and slowly shook his head, then he laughed his embarrassed Chinese laugh. 'We'll have to talk about that later,' he said.

The actual choice of the acupuncture sites turned out to be the most suitable for my diagnosis of liver disease, and everything was arranged for lowering the ascending liver Qi. The needles remained in place for fifteen minutes. Two rounds of treatment each consisting of eight sittings were agreed upon with the patient.

I found it unpleasant that all the doctors smoked in the presence of their patients. Chinese acupuncture doctors hold a cigarette in their left hand while they administer the needles with the right. The treatment rooms are not only full of stale smoke, but they are also rather cold. One could not only see cigarette smoke issuing from their mouths, but also their breath! Here, there is no such thing as central heating, neither in homes nor in the clinics. Fortunately, we were not here during the winter; today was 11 May.

In China, patients only undress to a certain degree, and often reveal very little skin for treatment. They do not give the impression of being particularly smart; on the contrary, they are rather dirty in general. Few of the women are properly washed, made up or perfumed. All of them have a stale body odour. They don't stink in the European sense, but nevertheless they do not smell pleasant either. We Europeans smell different anyway, but in comparison with my German or my Swiss patients, who always turn up well dressed and well groomed, the difference is like that between night and day.

The older doctor, who regularly practised at the Hua-Dong, did not possess good needle technique. He placed his needles superficially and was not at all sure of his choice of locations. He often stood in front of a patient for more than ten minutes and just rubbed his forehead with his fingertips. Moreover, his hand shook, and he was at least sixty years old. Our teachers at the college had a much better technique. At least, this was how it seemed to me. They placed their needles deeper and often they did this pretty roughly.

A female patient who worked as a typist was next. She had trouble with her stomach after meals. Her tongue was pale and swollen and had many grooves in the middle. Her pulse was weak and fine. The diagnosis was 'emptiness of the spleen and stomach'. She was asked not to eat cold meals or take cold drinks. Only four needles were used to treat her on her belly. Moxa burning was applied to the area around the navel. This procedure also lasted for about fifteen minutes.

Then a patient entered who had a sciatic problem, and this time the diagnosis of 'meridian illness' was correct. The kind of acupuncture applied was the same as we use in Europe: points on the back and in the hollow of the knee were punctured. Then there was a woman with lumbago. She worked in a restaurant. Here, a treatment was applied to her back. Another patient came in who worked in a laundry and who had pain in the back. I immediately thought of kidney weakness, but only two needles were administered to the left and right of his spinal column. They were stimulated by an electric current transmitted via a wire, so that the attached needles hopped up and down in the muscle of the back to the rhythm of the electrical impulse.

The last patient was a young woman suffering from morning diarrhoea between 5 and 6 o'clock. She had brought her X-ray photos with her, and from these one could see that she had a dropped stomach, which hung down into the pelvis. From the other X-rays one could see that one of her kidneys had suffered the same fate. Such general ptosis of the inner organs is quite commonly met with in China and is due to chronic undernourishment. According to Chinese medicine, this is the result of a weakness of the spleen, which favours the sinking of all other organs. Our western medicine then refers to this as gastroptosis associated with the dislocation of the kidney, but Chinese medicine considers it to be one unified disease. Taking the pulse or looking at the tongue or even examining the patient directly cannot confirm displacements such as these. In the West, the X-ray is the only reliable means of establishing a correct diagnosis.

I was pleased about this possibility and mentioned it to Dr Kang, and he was glad about my praise. The young woman received four needles and all the points were then warmed by using a burning moxa cigar. Since this was a chronic disease and quite dangerous, she was to come to the hospital every two days. She had already undergone needle treatment somewhere in Shanghai without success and had been at that time obliged to attend a sitting once a week. Because of this, the intervals between appointments had now been shortened.

As we went down the stairs together, Dr Kang remained at my side and remarked: 'Your diagnosis in the migraine case wasn't wrong; we'll have to talk about that.'

He nudged me in the ribs with his sharp elbow and said quietly: 'Ni shi Zhong-Yi! You are a Chinese doctor!'

This meant something like: 'What are you doing here as a Chinese doctor?'

In view of the stiffness and reserve so common in China, I was astonished by this indirect gesture of recognition.

A European Patient in Shanghai

Back in the hotel room I found an Achille complaining loudly of backache. This was so intense that he could hardly do anything to help himself. I was confronted with a sick European surgeon.

'Do you want me to treat you?' I asked.

'What? Do you think I'm going to submit myself to these shit methods! We've happily tortured enough poor devils in the clinic today!'

But his pain was so great that he let me at least examine him. He turned over to lie on his belly.

'Pain on pressure applied to the sacroiliac joint, on the spinous processes and in the paravertebral area.'

'What do you suggest?'

'I'll place three needles on each side, the Shen Shu, the Wei Zhong and the Zhi Bian. You know these already from your lessons.'

He agreed and I went off to get needles and swabs.

Just at this moment there was a knock at the door. It was Dr Gan with the female professor who had taught us needle and burning techniques. They arrived in the company of three interpreters.

'We have heard that Dr Haubensack is in pain,' they said.

'How the hell do they know that?' Achille asked me.

'They've got the whole room wired up,' I answered, 'I've already told you that.'

Had our hosts really bugged our place?

Dr Gan said at this point, 'It is not a good thing for Mr Rompard to treat you, because he's not allowed to practise medicine on his own here in China. But we'd be glad to help you.'

Achille had already taken all his clothes off and lay ready for treatment on the bed. The five Chinese stood wide-eyed, since Chinese were not in the habit of disrobing so completely.

'They all want to admire your charming Alsatian bum.'

While Achille laughed at this into his pillow, Gan had already very quickly placed his needle about four centimetres into Achille's buttocks. He then proceeded to set another needle into the Wei Zhong at the back of his knee without Achille feeling the need to utter even a murmur of protest. Gan then added the Da-Chang-Shu.

Finally, cupping glasses were placed over the needles, after which the Chinese delegation then withdrew, leaving me with the job of taking out the needles and removing the cupping glasses. Apparently, one didn't need any medical qualifications for this task. When the needles had been removed, Achille said he was completely free of pain.

After eating, we went off to try on our new suits that we had had cut by the tailor at the Friendship Store. Achille felt so well that he seemed to be walking on clouds. His pain had vanished completely and he could really fly – if he wanted to, he said.

'I felt exactly like that after receiving my first acupuncture treatment in Hong Kong,' I said. 'That's why I wanted to learn the technique myself one day.'

'Really?' Achille was exultant as we went along. 'I've seldom felt so well as I do this evening – absolutely free of ballast!'

I hoped that after this positive experience, Achille would think better of Chinese medicine.

Preparation for an Initial Examination

Typical of Chinese acupuncture is the fact that it is based on unacceptable theories as far as western medical people are concerned, and yet at the same time it can bring forth quite remarkable therapeutic results. Of course, one can proceed from the standpoint that such impressive effects will give way one day to a scientifically plausible explanation. On the other hand, the reservation lingers on as to how such powerful medical phenomena could last so long without much more than a pretty threadbare theoretical basis. At the academy, work proceeded from the ancient bases of assumption taken from the *Huang-Di Nei-Jing*. Any scientific foundation for these seemed to play second fiddle, and in this I found my long-held convictions confirmed while I was there that China's form of healing desperately needs modern western medicine in order to be at all understood and to be rendered reliable. Such fanciful diagnoses as 'emptiness of the stomach and the spleen' and 'emptiness of the kidney Qi' are just untenable for a western physician.

One of our students, an elderly doctor, had fallen ill. It was the old Syrian, the cardiologist who was sick due to the all-pervading cigarette smoke and the sticky air of the teaching rooms while we were studying the human body model with its lines and points on the surface. He had not been seen at meals since then. In the preceding days he had appeared paler and paler and last Sunday he seemed very depressed and asked me whether I was afraid of the immanent examinations. He said he had proved himself a terrible flop in all his tests up to now.

I told him that, to be sure, I was anxious at times, because one didn't know what kind of tasks and questions would be asked. At the last evening meal at which he was present again, he banged on the table with both fists several times so that the crockery and cutlery protested. The personnel rushed to the table. Such behaviour was very unusual here. One simply did not bang on tables. It could be that a study trip such as this led to a huge amount of physical stress for elderly people, and our Syrian colleague was simply not up to it. His state could also have been due to the political fuss, the mystery mongering, the primitively equipped clinic and the generally substandard medical facilities.

The climatic change alone presented a certain challenge to the body, and on top of this there was the need to adapt to the kind of food here. Above all, there was the need, too, to learn and to work. Achille and I, for example, sat for two hours every night to recapitulate what had been presented to us during lessons, and apart from this, he and I continued each day to study some new Chinese characters.

Where we could, we brightened things up a bit with Tsing-Tao beer and the wretchedly sweet red wine, whereas our interpreters and the majority of our teachers abstained completely from alcohol. One of our women teachers intimated to Achille in reference to his back pain of the previous day that he was far too fat, and that was why he was prone to the attacks he was suffering from. I mentioned that we Europeans were used to eating more substantial food than the Chinese and for this reason tended to put on weight. All of us were getting far too little exercise, whereas at home we were used to playing tennis or golf and to going hiking or skiing in the winter; we could also go swimming or walking every day, and there was nothing of that here. As proof of all this, I pinched the fat on my body which had accumulated in the one and half months I had been in China. This was the result of lack of body training, but was also due to our unhealthy food, which was becoming worse each day that went by. It is interesting to note that one just does not see obese Chinese with loads of stored fat on their arms and behinds. This is not surprising, since the Mainland Chinese get much less to eat than we do. For this reason, they are often ill during the winter. They have little immunity against infectious diseases, and they nourish themselves almost exclusively from rice and a bit of boiled cabbage three times a day. They can only eat meat once in a while, and even then there is not much of it to go round, and certainly not enough for proper nourishment. I once heard somewhere that a family of four living in Shanghai receives one egg per person per month. That is pretty depressing when one thinks that we as 'guests of the state' were receiving everything that could be placed on a table, and that at the reception dinner we were treated to a sumptuous banquet. At midday, we were allowed to eat to satiety and we were always served with beer, coffee and tea. This underlined the high level of hospitality bestowed on us, despite all the rigours of political and medical organisation that were involved.

Achille told me that he had come to China because his wife had urged him for months to at least visit this foreign country and there learn the arts of acupuncture, since, after all, he had received a governmental allowance to do so. And again, this new therapy was the talk of the town and a veritable sensation in Europe. The majority of his colleagues in France, the surgeons, orthopaedic specialists and neurologists, had turned down the offer, because they feared that their absence from work would lead them to suffer financial loss. Four months in China would mean a third less of their normal income, and in such a case, a European doctor can find himself in budgetary difficulties. Our respective governments paid for the flight and for the stay in China, though they did not compensate us for loss of income. If her husband, as the only doctor in Lorraine, didn't take advantage of this unique offer, then he was simply stupid, Mrs Haubensack concluded. He would never have the opportunity again. So it was that, with a heavy heart, Dr Haubensack undertook the long journey to China. Perhaps he could indeed help his patients in Nancy by applying acupuncture to relieve their pain instead of having to prescribe pain-relieving drugs in cases where he could not operate, such cases always leaving him somewhat irritated at not being able to do so.

Since his experience the previous day with acupuncture, Achille had taken opportunity to study particularly hard. Whenever he could, he painted Chinese characters, and he urged me at every turn when it came to a new idea to give him the Chinese character for it. But we were not that far along yet. I had to make it clear to him that many concepts and ideas that we had come across in the college lessons were in fact bad western translations of the Chinese original. He should go out into the street and into shops and elsewhere to work the meaning of things out for himself. This would be a great step forward for him.

For the final examination we had to learn 160 acupuncture points, and that for a beginner is far too many. However, I knew more than two thirds of these and used them regularly in my practice at home, and so for this reason needed only to learn a few more; the rest would be recapitulation.

It was also interesting to learn that between the various schools in Beijing, Shanghai and Canton there were certain differences to be observed. Some schools had apparently introduced new points and given them new names. Those in the know in Shanghai laughed about them and told us that these so-called new acupuncture points had long been referred to in the *Nei-Jing*. The point, Yao-Qi, for example, is to be found beneath the coccyx for the school in Beijing and Shanghai, but for the academy in Canton it lies under the spinous process of the fourth sacral vertebra. For the schools in Beijing and Shanghai, this point is identical with the point Yao-Yu, a point on the Du-Mai vessel which is already explained in the *Nei-Jing*. But a colleague in

Canton regarded this point as one newly discovered by his Canton academy. This was something that greatly amused the other Chinese schools of acupuncture.

Learning Tai-Ji-Quan

Yesterday, we had our first lesson in Tai-Ji-Quan, which had been prescribed for us because a number of colleagues had complained that we were getting insufficient exercise. A Tai-Ji teacher came to the hotel in the evening and we practised on one of the roof terraces. In addition to me, the Persian, the Swiss surgeon, Walo Sifferlin and the organiser, Lao Lu, who wanted to 'oil his old bones' so that they could function as they once did, took part in the exercises. Our teacher then treated us to a clumsy introductory speech that worked itself up to include what Mao Tse-tung once said about the need for these exercises to be done each day to maintain health, and also referred to their considerable medical value. Then he proceeded to show us what to do.

I noticed that this man had an enormously long fingernail on the little finger of his right hand. This meant that he was exonerated from all physical work. Such a long nail is to be seen in the case of other Asian people. He first demonstrated how we had to stand for the execution of Tai-Ji. There followed balancing exercises, and then, in conclusion, the first steps. We were to come along four times a week at five thirty after our work in the clinic and practise together for an hour. There were two interpreters present; one interpreted while the other just stood around looking rather embarrassed. Towards the end of the lesson, no doubt inspired by our clumsy efforts to copy our teacher, he took part in the exercises as well.

Looking for Partners and Marriage in Modern China

One evening I was with Adrienne Coningk and Herr Gröber in a Szechuan-style restaurant in Nanking Road. We placed our bikes against a tree and were immediately surrounded by a group of people who just stood and stared at us. Above all, they were fascinated by Adrienne's bright blonde hair. I placed myself boldly in front of this impertinent mob and stared back at them just as cheekily. One of them began to laugh. We went up to the second floor. Here there were a number of groups of Chinese engaged in eating, and this in such a way that beer and mineral water simply flowed from the bare brown wooden tables. The remains of food, together with bones and fish bones, were strewn around on the table and on the floor. There were no tablecloths or serviettes here. The Chinese are in the habit of shoving food into their mouths with chopsticks, chewing it there for a while and then spitting it out onto the table in order to look at it critically. Then they put the bolus back into their mouths again, retrieve it from there once more with their fingers and at the same time chatter loudly with their neighbours at table, an activity which is now and then punctuated by belching and long, penetratingly loud farts. The ancient Dutch painters would have had a whale of a time here, Adrienne remarked. We stood considering whether we would not be better off in a separate room, since the spectacle of Chinese at meal was not conducive to stimulating our appetite.

As soon as we had entered the restaurant, those present immediately let their chopsticks fall and gawped, open-mouthed, at us without saying a word. They looked like so many fish come up for air in a large aquarium. Herr Gröber sought to make it clear to the personnel that we would like a room to ourselves, but was told that everything was occupied. We were asked to take a seat at a table where a man and his wife were sitting, and this we did. I tried to pull a chair over to seat myself, but was not allowed to; the waiter had to fulfil this function. The couple at the table were friendly and greeted us with 'Nimen hao'. They were interested above all in the beautiful Adrienne.

We received beer first of all and then came various Szechuan dishes onto the table, Szechuan rice, Szechuan beef and Szechuan crab. We talked to Gröber about Chinese medicine, and he talked about his experiences with the Chinese. He lived with two Chinese students together in one room in a students' hostel. One of these students was a member of the Communist Party, the other not. The party member always had essential things to do and was often invited out, had more money to spend, and made sure that everyone else knew how important he was. The other student merely ran with the herd, like most folks here. Even among Chinese students there is such a thing as a new political class – namely, that comprising party members – although there is supposed to be no such thing as 'class'.

Adrienne asked how future marriage partners got to know each other. Gröber then told us that couples who wanted to marry often grew up in the same surroundings together or worked in the same place. If someone remained unmarried for too long, then the party intervened – meaning by this the people who control and observe everything that happens. If they feel that he or she must finally get married, then it will be organised. He will receive a free ticket to the cinema and next to him there will be a nubile young woman of the same age, anxious for matrimony. The rest is easy, say the organisers, and the party caters for every eventuality. As a modern, emancipated young European woman, Adrienne found the very idea appalling.

I mentioned that our women interpreters use their physical contact with us doctors to their advantage and often come near to touching us. They feel the natural warmth of the male and so to some extent make up for the erotic experience which is denied them. Gröber related that it was the same on buses. There, the young women voluptuously press their fullness close to the men, but more than this is not allowed.

For the most part, the laws pertaining to sexual abstinence are followed, very difficult though this is. Often enough they are impossible to conform to and then it happens that a Chinese woman gives birth to a child out of wedlock. She is immediately separated from the child, which is taken away from her, and she herself is sent off to a 'rehabilitation camp' where she will be subjected to hard daily work, and drilled in Mao's axioms on socially correct behaviour. When she leaves this kind of place, her only wish is to get away for ever from China, a 'home' which has brutally and shamefully robbed her of her human dignity.

Adrienne was frankly disgusted: 'If I had known this before, I wouldn't have come here,' she said.

Western Newspapers as 'Pornography'

One of our professors at the academy showed us a copy of the German *Stern* magazine. On the front cover there was a picture of a young woman in a bathing suit. In Europe, no one would have given the illustration a second thought. The effect of such photos has long been numbed. However, here it has a shock effect on people. Inside, there were other naked or half-naked young ladies to be admired. Our professor seemed to be entirely unaffected – or gave us that impression. He gazed stony-faced at the pictures, the corner of his mouth pulled down in contempt, and yet he could not for the life of him turn his head away from looking at them. Indeed, he seemed to be hypnotised. His face, however, only registered pure derision.

This immediately reminded me of a schoolmate of mine at secondary school who came from an ultra-Catholic background and who, to us, strangely enough, was a bigot. It was an odd situation, because nobody could take his specious piety seriously. He never laughed at our jokes, for example, could never find a grin for our frivolities, our obscene insinuations (we were about 15 or 16 years old) that made up the essential stuff of our adolescent conversation at that time. He would pull a disdainful face very similar to that worn by our Chinese acupuncture professor, with one corner of the mouth screwed down in scorn. This went on for some time, perhaps for a year, until one day we were in the school yard eating what was called 'school meals'. On this occasion, our friend had filled his mouth full of pea soup, soup which he could not swallow because it was too hot. We were busy with our obscenities as usual, in such a way that he had to hear everything we said. We joked and made lewd remarks without letting up. He heard everything, of course, but kept a straight face. Then, suddenly, he simply exploded with laughter. We noted with satisfaction that, behind the façade of pious rectitude, he had secretly appreciated everything that had been said. He simply could not hold back any longer, and without warning, like the eruption of a mighty volcano, he lost his unctuous composure. In doing so, he unloaded a mouthful of pea soup, enriched with sausage pieces, into the air in a high arc to land as a green stream straight onto the grey jacket and white flannels of the good Professor Fidi, who happened to be dining next to him.

Now, of course, we were right royally amused – in the first place by the sudden change in our companion, but no less by the damage done to our teacher's apparel. It was to be a therapy for our schoolmate and had a permanent effect on him. He was cured for ever of his ecclesiastical hypocrisy, but our teacher harboured a grudge against us for the spoiled garments. Our classmate was cured of his bigotry. He became a member of our frivolous group and in the end indulged in dirty jokes himself. In fact, we had unknowingly administered a kind of effective psychotherapy on him.

Here in the middle of Mao's socialist kingdom, I must say that I never saw a party member laugh uninhibitedly. The laugh that frees the soul was forbidden. There was no release for the locked-up socialist unconscious 'id' of the Chinese people. Anyone making jokes or caricatures that ridiculed the party or its organisation, or that derided the stilted bombast of Chinese social structure, was brutally punished. All manner of creativity was therefore nipped in the bud. From the medical aspect – that is, from the point of view of psychological hygiene – this seemed to me to be very alarming. Every day we saw oppression in the faces of our anxious, browbeaten patients and treated them for psychosomatic diseases which, for party reasons, could only be treated as physical illnesses. For this reason, many sick people here just could not be helped.

Whenever I had the rare opportunity to talk privately with a Chinese person, it was something of a windfall and was in any case forbidden. In such cases, I used the simplest of Chinese as a means of communication. Anyone who was dependent on an interpreter had absolutely no chance of hearing anything about the personal fate of an individual. Now and again I took the chance to get into personal conversation with patients at the clinic in order to learn more about them and their country.

In my luggage I had a book written by a psychiatrist from Latin America entitled *Psychotherapy for the Masses*. The author had often been invited to China to assess the situation of mental hygiene in the country. Apparently, he had never experienced anything of all the appalling horror we encountered each day here. The gnomes at the top had, it seems, successfully managed to hide from him all the poisonous elements of moral oppression in communist China's society.

Our severe moral critic of the *Stern* magazine was the same medical man, by the way, who had treated Achille Haubensack the other day in our room. As he turned his glance away in contempt from the offending pictures, an interpreter tore the magazine from his hands and lasciviously scanned the pages for more flesh. The doctor was then in no position to carry on a medical conversation with us, and was forever glancing over to the interpreter out of the corner of his eye. Noticing at last that he had finished, he in his turn tore the journal out of the other's hands and went through it with a glare of electrified intensity in order not to miss anything that might catch his lecherous interest.

The difficulty of treating patients in China hangs together with this tradition of affected moralising. That day, for example, we had a prudish female patient suffering from a post-operative problem of the uterus. She removed her dress sufficiently enough to reveal a small area of skin around the navel. However, to treat her it would be necessary to go a little further below. There then began a millimetre-by-millimetre struggle to remove her underclothes to facilitate proper investigation of the problem. The woman put up strong resistance to this. However, without the removal of her underclothes, no endeavours on our part would be able to help her, not with the best will in the world. Moreover, it was intended to administer moxa treatment, a procedure which, in this fully clothed situation, would have committed the poor, pain-racked woman to the flames!

We experienced something similar at the academy. Here, every male acupuncture dummy was covered with a small loincloth, so that no one may know what was underneath the cloth and get the idea that there in fact are two sexes. When I asked why the acupuncture dolls were always male and why one couldn't use a pretty Chinese girl as an acupuncture model in lectures from time to time, I received grim looks from teachers and interpreters alike, who refused to translate my question. I had clearly gone too far with my enquiry.

The classical 'copper man', the Tong-Ren of Wang Wei-Yi, was also a man, Professor Shi explained. And that's why. Everything had a historical origin, and tradition was always respected here in China.

'That's not true!' I objected. 'Mao, the great Chairman, did away with many traditions – the teaching of Confucius was one of them.'

I should not really have said such a thing, because our teacher was in danger of losing face.

'That's quite another matter,' the interpreter said. 'Mao has decreed that it be so, Mao is our Great Helmsman! His is the last word and argument.'

Apparently one twists the so-called revolutionary logic around to suit such a situation.

I pursued the issue nevertheless: 'But Mao Tse-tung doesn't think much of this tradition, as we all know. He always talks of men and women being equal and having the same rights. Would it not be fitting now to document this in the teaching of acupuncture and, in addition to the "Nan Tong-Ren", the male "copper man" doll, also to equip the academy with a "Nü Tong-Ren", a female "copper woman" dummy?' With this comment it was quite clear that I had overstepped the mark again. The Chinese teachers left the room in silence – and to a man!

Achille asked Dr Kang whether during the examination we might not be allowed to undress ourselves so that we can demonstrate the acupuncture points with their complicated Chinese names on our own bodies. Kang noted the ulterior motive behind this request and answered his question with a tight face by saying that, yes, this would be possible, but we would only be allowed to bare our arms and legs, not any other part of the body.

Interpreters' Wrong Renderings

Today, a discussion arose at the university on the correct definition of concepts in Chinese medicine that were to be rendered into French. A topic of debate was the concept of phlegm, 'Tan', 痰, mucus. Our interpreters translated that from their dictionaries as 'sputum'. But the pictograph 'Tan' means something different in Chinese, and indeed much more than mere 'mucus'. It happens to be a large, comprehensive, pathological dimension from which, incidentally, many hundreds of varying diseases can arise. Adnan Kirinin, our black colleague from Cameroon, mentioned that the ideograph was constructed from the radical component 疒, which means to lie on a bed or to be sick, and from yan, 炎, a rising flame or a burning fire. So Tan always indicates a quite serious condition of illness.

'From "Tan" a multitude of diseases come into being,' the appropriate passage from the *Su-Wen* thus reads.

I suggested transcribing the Chinese original only using Pin-Yin and then explaining it according to its Chinese medical meaning, so as to be sure not to need further translation. This suggestion met with general approval. This was necessary so as to avoid the translation being steered in quite another direction to the one originally intended. In this way, wrong western implications could be avoided. Western 'rationalisations' had the habit of totally deforming the original Chinese, with the consequence that they were completely incomprehensible.

During the whole of the lecture, the noise below us of shouting and tramping students learning acupuncture points their own way made itself felt. 'San Li Nei Ting Xue. Qu Chi He Gu Jie, Wei Zhong Pei Cheng Shan, Tai Chong Kun Lun Xue ...' These were the names of acupunture points that can be used jointly and combined in treating a patient.

Achille stuck his fingers in his ears. 'How can we study such a complicated matter in the midst of that terrible hubbub?' he lamented.

One of our female instructors came over and asked him what he had to complain about. 'It is much too noisy in the classroom,' he answered.

'Noisy?' she replied, ostensibly surprised. 'But it is very quiet in this room, isn't it?'

'No', said Achille, 'it's not!'

Then the woman quickly changed the subject. 'We Chinese teachers are usually modest and exert ourselves to make things easier for you to understand. In doing this, we are not anxious to be the only authority and so maintain that we are always in the right, but we really want you to learn.'

The instructor had been talking about the techniques using needle application and moxa burning. She felt that we would be able to discriminate between needle techniques used at home and those practised in Shanghai. In reply I told her that there was actually no such thing as a 'European needle technique'. I explained that up to now, techniques and theories of acupuncture in Europe have owed their accomplishment to the French school, and as a consequence good translation is lacking and for the most part is devoid of congruence with the original Chinese. There was nothing for it, therefore, I concluded, than to finally orientate ourselves with the original Chinese terms in order to arrive at all at serious training in Chen-chiu geared to Chinese medicine.

'Our interpreters were especially well trained to render the correct translation of each Chinese medical term to you,' the woman said.

I mentioned the problem to her that we had experienced earlier with the translation of 'Tan'.

'The dictionaries of our interpreters are absolutely reliable,' she said and walked away.

'At this point you can literally grasp the hermetic Great Wall which isolates us from understanding the Chinese,' Achille said to me.

'It's the same the other way round,' I added.

Our Tailors Show us the Revolutionary Cold Shoulder

Today I was in the Friendship Shop in order to collect a new white suit and a light grey one. After I had been satisfied with my first suit I had ordered these two in the hope of the same excellent workmanship as before. I was to be horrified, however, when I tried the new garments on. They looked as though I had been beaten up in them! Nothing fitted. The arms on one of the jackets were too long and the jacket itself hung to the kneecaps. It was clear that the work had been given to an inexperienced novice. This kind of thing happens. A revolutionary committee can, on occasion, regulate the work on suits. It was not for nothing that the tailor had to shut up shop after our visit and run off to the Revolutionary Committee to report all that had been said and done. Here, we were not to be seen walking around in excellent attire. That was far too capitalistic.

These folks, I said to myself, *can't be the famous Far Eastern Shanghai tailors who are deemed to be the best in the world.* What I experienced was sloppy work. The material I had chosen was of the very best, and it had been ruined. A third suit that I had ordered did not sit either, neither top nor bottom, front nor back. It was clear that there was not the slightest interest in pleasing those whom the Chinese referred to as 'our foreign guests' or 'friends' with anything of quality. Why should what the Chinese themselves could not afford be given to others, to foreigners?

As soon as I appeared at the door, the tailor raised his piping voice from a room at the back of the shop and cried, 'Paper! Paper!'

He wanted to see the paper on which the contract had been written, otherwise he would send me back to the hotel without more ado to get this wretched piece of paper. This same drama had happened twice before.

'But you've known me now for three weeks!' I protested.

'No. Never seen you before!' he said, lying.

He pretended not to know me, although he himself had taken my measurements and personally seen me through several fittings. He was clearly uncomfortable about his lying and insincerity, and for this reason he cried out all the louder: 'Paper! Paper!'

I declined to take the new suits with me. The tailors refused to alter them anyway.

'Fit welly, welly well,' they kept saying like a machine.

'No, they don't fit well at all!' I complained, but to no avail. Exasperated, I threw the suits into the room and left without another word. I could see from their expressions that they knew full well how I felt. One of them laughed scornfully as I went out.

I feared I would have to write another letter to the ambassador in Beijing.

Contradiction and Unity

We saw patients today who had been previously treated by us. Some of them felt better, others not. It was something I was familiar with in my European practice.

I asked the young female professor who had been teaching us from the beginning about confirming pregnancy by taking the pulse. 'Yes,' she replied, 'it is indeed possible and even in the first days of pregnancy, and even before the first laboratory tests give a positive result. If the patient is healthy and not suffering from any pathological pulse changes brought about by illness, then confirmation can be given which is later confirmed by laboratory tests.'

This colleague, who was obviously versed in gynaecology, was of the opinion that laboratory investigation was more reliable than pulse diagnosis.

'Above all, one should already be acquainted with the patient – in other words, be familiar with her normal pulse before she becomes pregnant. Otherwise it is impossible to register a difference,' she said. 'The most certain way of ascertaining whether a patient is pregnant or not is to apply a combination of the western and the traditional Chinese medical methods.'

I was of the same opinion and based this conclusion on my experience gained from having worked as a gynaecological assistant and country doctor where, with the help of well-qualified midwives, I had guided and personally assisted at about a hundred births.

'I feel that in this area of pulse diagnostics one should also have had plenty of experience in modern midwifery and gynaecology,' I said in reply to my colleague's opinion, and she promptly agreed with me.

'Without this practical experience, it is impossible to say anything according to the tenets of traditional Chinese medicine. Mao Tse-tung realised this in saying, "All real knowledge stems from practical experience."'

After this, there was a discussion between the Chinese doctors who were present. Apparently, in China today there is a development within the social control organs – that is, the Communist Party members working on the growth of a modern Chinese state – concerning this.

This principal tendency throws up the following question: 'How can one still believe in all the superstitious hogwash which once was part of ancient China, a time when one believed in ghosts and spirits, in the influence of the heavens on human affairs, and in the influence of the dead who were always on the alert to subvert human activity?'

(By the way, many Chinese still believe in ghosts and spirits! But the party denies and contests it.)

For this reason, the communists turn up their noses at the decadent West where such things as parapsychology and spiritism, along with other psychological, pseudo-scientific perplexities are officially recognised. They go so far as to claim that the West will eventually go down as a result of these tendencies since, although it has achieved so much in modern technology, these achievements are not, in the long run, for the benefit of the people. This so-called liberalism is regarded here as extremely destructive for the 'revolutionary society', and for this reason, they say, it must be banned by law in order to protect the people.

To this I add my own comment that in Europe it is precisely Chinese medicine which has the taint of being spiritist or metaphysical and, above all, that suffers from being 'unscientific'. Up to now it has always been researchers at the edge of medical investigation in Europe who have concerned themselves with Chinese traditional medicine. Without these people, however, no one in Europe would know anything about acupuncture, for example. Even if such people had had the weirdest ideas about the subject, they were nevertheless the forerunners in founding Chinese healing methods in the West. And this was only possible because the western liberal states were open to new ideas.

Dr Kang then gave his explanation for this: '"The Law of Internal Contradiction" concerning all things is also "The Law of Unity" in all things and is in fact the most fundamental law of dialectical materialism.'

To this I objected, 'But that's exactly the ancient doctrine of Yin-Yang which has just been adapted to suit your dialectical materialistic thinking.'

'Well, we haven't created this idea,' he retorted. 'Mao Tse-tung, our great Helmsman, has made this clear to us Chinese, and he was right. Yin-Yang is the oldest law we have and stems from a society which, thousands of years ago, was a primitive, classless society, and for that reason, naturally, a communist one to which we have now returned. At that time, too, there was the Law of Contradiction in everything, and at the same time there was the Law of Unity of all things, and that was Ying-Yang.'

And then Professor Xiong gave me his commentary on his criticism already made on the metaphysical social evils in the West.

'Contradictory things show themselves in relation to the Unity of all things by their non-identity. As a consequence, they don't only exist in common, but can, like Yin and Yang, always change into their opposites. That's happened with you in the West as far as acupuncture and Chinese medicine is concerned. We see the final confirmation of the correctness of the teaching of our great chairman, Mao, in this.'

I was speechless at this. Then I retorted: 'Well, according to this, then, the Law of Contradiction could well end up one day working towards the opposite of material-dialectical thinking. In other words, your communist society today could, according the tenets of logic and the intrinsic nature of the law we speak of, convert the communist society into its direct opposite.'

All those present held up their hands in horror at this and looked around in the hope that no one had heard the conversation.

'That will never ever happen,' they said in choir, 'because we've reached our highest objective, the union of the Chinese masses.'

The pressure towards getting the Chinese to think along the same lines probably has ancient roots based on a concern with the theory of unity in the universe. It is a great pity, therefore, that today it has been turned in such a way as to be aligned with Marxist-materialist thinking. The idea of everyone thinking on the same lines is a very old Chinese concern. Added to this, the ideology of dialectical materialism has found a niche within it. It is never said aloud, but much of it originates in the teaching of Confucius. An example of its implication today is the modern subservience to the state and its dictates, the obsequious observance of the regulations decreed by the party, especially the monstrous laws concerned with sexual behaviour, although this, too, played a great role in ancient China. Another people, untouched by the moral dictums of a Confucius, would not tolerate them.

We can say, then, that the Chinese show a strong tendency towards infantilism. When someone puts up with anything dictated from above without resistance, then that, from the European point of view, demonstrates a lack of personal maturity. When one, further, like Mao Tse-tung, suggests that the most important event in the world is eating, that, too, from a psychoanalytical point of view, is the continuance of the small child's oral phase in which everything can be valued first by the tongue that receives nourishment and experiences how it tastes and how nourishing it is. A common form of greeting in China is illustrative of this: 'Chi-Fan-le? Have you eaten yet?' I always think of this when I hear the chopsticks clattering on the bowls and this greeting making its rounds while Chinese are at their meals.

From the point of view of Europeans, the Chinese are not yet quite grown up. This endurance of childish behaviour, this infantilism in psychoanalytic terms, is a regression, a return to an earlier stage of individual development. This is exactly what some people who emigrate here from Europe are looking for in the East. They are looking for a treacherous, cosy safety under the wings of some primordial father, or for the womb of a primordial mother, the 'Great Chairman' and his party, because they cannot survive in the rough and tumble of a capitalistic society. This is probably what happens in the first place, and I think automatically of the two German Maoist women of our acquaintance. In the long run, however, this is dangerous, because the individual gradually loses his or her powers of discrimination. Should these people ever return to Europe, their necessary re-integration into western society would be accordingly more difficult. Here in China, for example, they are impotent to show their teeth to their circumstances and fall all too easily into the dream of a 'heavenly, beautiful China'. As they do so, they remove themselves more and more from reality. Viewed psychopathologically, this is a neurotic development which is nothing less than a disease needing treatment.

Achille and I both believed that we were already going this way. The constant ideological pressure had changed us. Only through discussion and studying our Chinese characters were we keeping our heads above water and concentrating on that which we had come to seek and not yet found.

Along with this modern tendency in China, there are things which have remained intact within China's history and culture. One of these is the morning practice of Tai-Ji-Quan through which the Chinese experience what they call an 'absorption into the universe', or 'establishing a personal relationship with the rest of creation in space', by which, they say, 'heaven and earth are brought into harmony'. So it is that the old Chinese heaven still plays a role in their lives.

Chinese patience also hangs together with its ancient culture. And in addition to all this, there is acupuncture, Chen-chiu, which belongs to Chinese medicine in the form handed down to us. I just cannot get rid of the suspicion somehow that acupuncture is only being superficially and demonstratively exhibited to the West in its Communist Party political aspects. In such a case, China has something to offer to the world, something which interests everyone – namely, health – and it is this which is being cleverly exploited for political and cultural purposes. Suddenly, China is no longer a country plagued by ignorance and famine, sleeping behind an impenetrable Great Wall of silence. China unexpectedly has something to offer the rest of mankind. 'But what is that, precisely?' western medicine asks.

The pride of thousands of years of Chinese achievement stands at odds with the typical, irrational belief in the power of western medicine. There are any number of patients and doctors in China who aver that 'if we only had the wonderful resources of the West in terms of medicaments and methods of healing, there wouldn't be so much suffering and not many sick people'. There is no doubt about the fact that in the highly populated city of Shanghai there are literally hundreds of thousands of sick people.

With regard to my own experience of human suffering in Shanghai's clinics, I can only say the following to those who believe in the party system: 'If you had created a more human society in your midst than this faceless mass of human ants, then there wouldn't be so many cases of functional disturbance, pain due to cancer and psychologically conditioned organic dysfunction which is so particularly high in Shanghai where there is greater emotional and political pressure, and consequently a greater lack of individual freedom.'

The Chinese attitude to western medicine corresponds to the irrational expectations with regard to Chinese healing methods and acupuncture in the West. Apparently, human beings need these idealistic concepts in order to project their unfulfilled wishes onto something unknown, something which, in this case, quickly loses its fascination when one begins to view it rationally and critically in daily practice.

Looked at from the social point of view and using the Law of Internal Contradiction of Things, we could say that as far as the relation of China to the West is concerned, the West is very individualistic. We research and analyse relationships so that we can personally see through them and understand them, and in doing so we necessarily separate ourselves from the mass of humanity. In communist China, the opposite is true. There is hardly a trace of individualism. There, one has forgotten, or has been forced to forget by the party, that every illness is in the very first place an extremely personal, individual matter, and this is confirmed in the ancient Chinese scripts on the human subject. According to them, medicine begins with an understanding of Shen, 神, the innermost part of a human being, and, along with it, with an understanding of the universal order. But all this is regarded as so much old-fashioned superstition in Mao's kingdom. The character Shen 神, when properly translated, means 'witness to the cosmic order'. But who knows of these things today? The Maoistic cosmos, which has created unity, is founded on material masses, on an anonymous, frequently chaotic and completely opaque assemblage of heterogeneous individual human beings who have no voice of their own. Mao's concept is finally out of touch with reality, itself an unconsidered metaphysical idea, because it insists on ignoring the essential kernel of a human being, the 'I', the Self or the personality.

Good medicine closely hangs together with the innate constitution of a patient, the Jing, 精, his or her internal essence. This essence is the essence of a patient's personal life. From these two, Shen, 神, and Jing, 精, arise blood, 血, and Qi, 氣, where the last two characters symbolise the individual life force, and play such an important part in needle therapy. This can only be realised within a humanistic state. Communist China offers hardly any opportunity at the moment for this to be unfolded. The violent appropriation of China's great tradition of healing by its communist rulers in Beijing might well go down in medical history as one of the greatest deformations of truth ever known.

For this reason, Chinese medicine on the mainland is a kind of paradox, because it is here that one is trying to dissolve the individual in the mass. There is no longer any logic in this 'new' medicine, but simply an acceptance at one go of the larger relationships of the system while at the same time trying to shove its practical applications into the foreground. To effect this display, the men in power are obliged to manipulate and falsify the whole to make it fit into the political armour of the Marx–Engels–Mao doctrine, since otherwise it would have no *raison d'être*. At least this is true in the case of acupuncture. There is hardly anyone here who is familiar with the ancient medical texts. This is the case in the clinics, where exact diagnoses are just never on the agenda, and where one merely scans the patient for a superficial set of symptoms to fit into a general picture of the illness, and where, further, needles are placed more or less at random in the hope that the healing processes will somehow, sometime take place. Then it can happen, as it did that morning, that one Chinese doctor will place his needles and, at the same time, another doctor present will whisper to a colleague that he does not agree at all with what is going on and that he would tackle the problem quite differently!

If I had then asked this doctor whether his method was better than the other, I would have receive the answer to the effect that, well, perhaps not, but one can approach this kind of disturbance from different angles. In other words, one is consistent in not giving an honest, direct answer. Is this what is meant by the 'Law of Contradiction at Work in All Things'? A lucid 'choice of method' or a consistent treatment directed towards achieving a clear objective is simply not to be found here. All this vagueness, however, can be well categorised in the fuzzy, undefined thinking of the communist Chinese.

But shouldn't we be a bit more careful in our judgement? It could just be that this vagueness, this chaotic Chinese picture of the universe fits the bill as it is, rather than our all too frequently imposed unnatural western order in the matter of understanding and scientific perception. In our medicine, of course, this hazy thinking does not correspond in any way to the precise picture we have of the human organism and its functions. But then, is western medicine a science at all? Does it not use the most varied of methods to reach its objectives, including the scientific? How does science tie up with such things as psychoanalysis or medical hypnosis? Why is it not possible for modern medicine to apply the thinking behind the ancient Chinese texts?

Here, new physics or quantum physics might show us the proper way to understand Chinese medicine and Chen-chiu better and in a new scientific light and framework.

A Political Cause of Illness

I had noticed that many Chinese patients were quite well disposed to us, and that, in the morning, they greeted us in the friendliest way when they entered the treatment room. This was especially the case when we had treated them before; they then accepted us as their doctors and allowed us to use the needle and moxa burning without demur. I liked to talk to them about personal things, something which the interpreters quietly frowned upon.

'You're not here to talk to the patient, but to treat her,' they warned me.

'The one is impossible without the other', I retorted, but they contradicted me.

'In a Marxist organised clinic,' they replied, 'that's not only possible, but common practice. The masses are to be treated by their doctors without a lot of gossip.'

Yesterday afternoon, I arrived at Hua-Dong Hospital about three quarters of an hour before my Chinese colleagues with their interpreters came along. I encountered a pale patient, crouched and withdrawn into himself, waiting in front of the treatment-room door. I knew him from previous treatments and asked him whether he felt better. He shook his head. I invited him to come in, fetched his documents from the pile lying ready and discovered that he was 28 years old, an engineer and married. According to the accompanying

X-rays, he was suffering from gastritis, and he was affected, too, by frequent migraine attacks.

He could speak a little English and I tried to get along in that language. I asked him whether he had any personal troubles and his face darkened.

'What's the matter?' I asked.

Falteringly, he told me that he had great personal problems. He had married a young woman who once lived in the same street, and so he had known her a long time. After study he could find no work in Shanghai, and on the party's order had to move to the Mongolian border and was even obliged to live there as this was the only place where he could find work. The young woman, his future wife, accordingly applied to the local party authorities for permission to follow him. This was granted and she moved north to join him. Up there, they were married immediately, since there they are not as strict with young people there as they are in other parts of the country.

Shortly after this, however, he was accorded a post in Shanghai which he had to accept against his will because the party ordered him to do so. He therefore returned to Shanghai, but his wife did not receive permission to return. In all probability she would have to remain on the Mongolian border for ever, alone for the rest of her life. And he would be here in Shanghai, he said miserably. The reason for this predicament was that many thousands of similar cases had already applied to return to Shanghai and his beloved wife had been placed right at the end of the list of applicants. Life up in the north, he added, was much harder and much more primitive than here in the city. He felt that it had been a great sacrifice on the part of his wife to make the application to go north and now he felt guilty for her unhappiness. He broke into tears at saying this. I had never seen a Chinese weeping before.

'No,' I said, 'it's your damned Communist Party which is guilty, not you.'

He was greatly shocked at this remark and whispered, 'Oh Doctor, you mustn't say such things!'

I told him that it was this situation that was the cause of his present condition, but that kind of thing was of no interest to the people here, either party bosses or doctors.

When the interpreters and Chinese colleagues arrived, they looked at me suspiciously.

'Have you treated him?'

'No,' I answered.

'What were you speaking to him about?' That's what interested them most.

'We talked about Shanghai weather, about his illness and about international friendship with the peoples of the world,' I said. The patient nodded readily in agreement. Even after twenty sittings, our acupuncture treatment brought him no relief.

My diagnosis in this case was not 'meridian disturbance', 'syndrome problems' or something of that sort, but I merely wrote in the report: 'Conversion of a mental condition into a physical illness.' It was in fact a typical psychosomatic illness.

I was greatly tempted to write: 'A severe illness of the autonomous nervous system brought on by Marxist–Maoist dialectic – that is, party-political contempt for human beings.'

The fact that this young man had been allowed to marry the wife of his choice in inner Mongolia had been a great exception to the general rule, which is that if people here want to marry, they have to live for six months or a whole year together, but they are not allowed to produce children. After this initial period, they are separated for between eight and ten years. They are sent to areas far apart from one another, so that they are not under any circumstances able to see each other during this time. When the 'couple' are at least thirty-five years of age, they will be allowed to marry and then they may produce one child. But only one! As a consequence, these people are exposed to enormous sexual tension. This leads to situations where young female students at a university never risk going into a room where there are several young males, because they fear being immediately attacked. That kind of thing is not infrequent here. We noticed something of the sort among our female interpreters. They never entered a room, for example, in which there might be one or several men.

The Shanghai newspapers and TV broadcasters had a lot to say about our visit in a TV presentation. They knew where we came from and who we were. We were allowed by our patients to touch their bodies, to look at their tongues and feel their respective pulses in diagnosing illness. I had the feeling that the needle combination was often put together according to a scheme. One day I asked old Dr Ou-Yang whether the course of the body vessels and the other concepts of Chinese medicine played a decisive part in it.

'Yes, they do,' he said, 'they play a great role. From these concepts, everything else is derived.'

We seldom saw this, though, in practice. We merely noted that our teachers stuck their heads together from time to time, 'ummed' and 'aahed' a little and then whispered acupuncture structures' names to each other. Then one would name this point and another that, and soon the recipe was ready. I don't know whether this was essentially as superficial as it looked.

But on the other hand, one thing seemed clear, and that was that many a medical man here used his needles in an 'Off we go' technique. They chose their points and body structures quite at random, sometimes according to their experience, and only on rare occasions did they proceed correctly if we were to take the classical rules of acupuncture technique into consideration.

Dr Kang intimated to me today that he personally felt that Chinese medicine was much better than modern western medicine. That's why he became a Chinese doctor. In the main, he said, he managed very well with its methods. He used western techniques in very few cases.

'Have you really understood western medicine?' I asked him. He looked at me quizzically.

'Our old Chinese physicians didn't know anything about western medicine either,' he replied, 'and they developed a means of healing which brings western doctors to China in hordes. Why, do you think?'

Why indeed? There must be something lacking in our western system of medicine up to the present day, I thought to myself, but said nothing. This Dr Kang could not have imbibed much from western medicine in a three-year course of study. The question was, could he attend satisfactorily to an injury, for example, or hold a consultation shortly after a woman's conception and see the whole thing through to birth? Could he read an ECG or an X-ray and draw logical conclusions from it? Did he know anything of the principles of modern pharmacology or the principles of prescription? Did he know anything about anatomy? Was he indeed a doctor at all in the comprehensively educated, western sense of the word?

Despite that, here he was my teacher, and, according to Chinese etiquette, one could not be allowed to criticise one's teacher. One had simply to listen.

V

Off to Fu-Dan University

On the following Sunday, we went into town with our respective cameras, constantly surrounded by a horde of Chinese who followed us like hungry birds, gawking at us and laughing at us as we went along. Children skipped around us like little apes. Everyone was highly amused by the most trivial of things. Adults here behave very much like children do in Europe. I asked myself whether it would be at all possible to govern such a people without a strict educational and disciplinary regimen. They would do nothing of their own accord, merely sit in the sun and perhaps do a little gymnastics or allow themselves to be duped and drowned out by loud music.

Yes, in former times this race was an industrious one which had made the most remarkable discoveries and which had gone down in history as part of the world's scientific development.

As individuals, the Chinese are not uncongenial, and they are really quite friendly when one talks to them. But in terms of how they regard us there is also something about them that is on the lookout for sensation, something akin to that which visitors to a zoo bring with them when they look through the bars of cages at the cooped-up animals. It is in fact a mixture of curiosity and fear.

In the afternoon I rode over to Fu-Dan university on my bike, and in so doing lost my way a couple of times. I had no plan of the city, since there is no such thing here. So I had to ask the way and cycled by quite a number of picturesque places. The buildings were very Chinese in character, meaning that they were very untidy, with heaps of dirt before their front doors on which hens picked and scratched. Washing was pulled on lines across the street and people sat in front of their houses playing cards.

After half an hour I managed to reach the university, which was pretty far away from the centre, surrounded by little country houses and small huts and vegetable patches. Here, too, goats, hens, pigs and other animals wandered about over the street, but the air was much cleaner than in Shanghai's city centre. I wanted to ride through the gate to the university, but the porter stopped me.

I had then to fill out a long questionnaire: Name? Profession? Nationality? Who did I want to see? What kind of personal relationship did I have with the person I wanted to visit at the university? What was the purpose of my visit? To which unit did I belong, and what was I doing in China? This was filled in in duplicate, the porter retaining one copy and handing me the other. The porter then showed me the way to the house I wanted to visit. Once there, I was obliged to sign my name to indicate my presence at a kind of reception area and present my questionnaire. The woman there was pleasant; apparently she was used to such visits. She pushed my bike in front of her into the house and was generally helpful.

I found the German sinology student I had come to see, Willibald Gröber, who lived on the first floor. He shared his apartment with two Chinese men, both university students like him. The room was gloomy, and after dark it had become very cold. He showed me a couple of books in Chinese which he was currently studying.

We did not stay long in these rather inhospitable circumstances in which, by the way, Gröber had been housed over the last two years, but decided to visit a nearby restaurant. However, when we got there, it was too late for an evening meal, and so we got nothing to eat. Not content with this situation, I took him to the Da-Shan Hotel. Before I could actually leave the university, however, I was again required to sign to the effect that I had left the premises officially, as it were, and state when and where and with whom, for the benefit of the person responsible for the residential block. Gröber, too, had to do the same. Only then were we allowed to leave the university premises. I found all this red tape particularly humiliating for a western visitor like myself. Anyway, we ate well in the hotel as a kind of consolation.

A First Examination

There was an intermediate examination today for us doctors. We had already got up at six in the morning in order to prepare the examination material. The examiners and the accompanying interpreters considered it a sort of celebration. Evidently, they took our examinations very seriously. Of course, proceedings were prefaced by the director of the institute giving a boring speech. Then we were divided into three groups.

I was placed in a group which included Achille, the two French ladies and the two Swiss. The Africans were placed in a group together with the Laotians and the Syrians and Persians. In terms of grade of difficulty, the examination was pretty simple as far as we were concerned.

Acupuncture questions were put to us and afterwards we were asked about the relationship of acupuncture points to the meridian lines in their complete lengths. In addition, we were asked to localise the course of these lines on the human body.

After we had shown that we knew a thing or two about these matters, the examination was felt to have run on satisfactory lines and everyone seemed content with its course. During it, however, there was no consideration given as to whether the knowledge that we had been supplied with was based on incorrect translations. I can see now in retrospect how thoroughly the Chinese professors regarded our training as providing us with the necessary qualifications to go on to treat Chinese patients in the various hospitals in the city. I must add to this, however, that when Chinese doctors are sent to Europe to work, their Chinese medical examination is not regarded as adequate qualification; they have to pass another examination recognised in European countries before being allowed to practise there or in the USA. It is otherwise impossible for them to practise medicine, they just cannot undertake the job and its responsibilities.

These implications were now being demonstrated to us in reverse, so to speak. The Chinese insist that 'you will have to take a further examination here in China before being allowed to practise in this country'. Certainly, from the Chinese point of view, there is the ulterior desire to check the effectiveness of their teaching methods and the quality of their interpreters.

Finally, they wanted to know whether we had used our time sensibly for study or whether we had merely spent it shopping and drinking coffee in the city.

Dr Kang did most of the questioning and was interpreted by Xiao Gu (Miss Gu). In the course of my questioning, I explained the relationship between the pericardium and the heart, which he found plausible.

In typically Beijing style, the interpreter strictly insisted that I separate the teaching material learned during the course and as had been previously prescribed. It irritated her to see that here and there I reserved my own opinion on matters. Individual opinion here is not desired; one is required to keep to the prevalent opinion of the 'masses', otherwise, it was very likely that, as a Chinese doctor, one would be sent into the countryside as a deviationist or counter-revolutionary or be reprimanded or disciplined in some unpleasant way or other. Anyone stepping out of Mao's line is not considered 'revolutionary' in the sense he demanded.

And then there is a peculiar attitude in the Far East to higher education and studying at a university. Students are just endlessly copying and repeating the matters they are supposed to learn. No deeper discussions with professors are permitted, and a view or an opinion of one's own is considered very bad manners. How, then, can someone really study a field of knowledge in terms of developing a personal and sincere understanding?

On the other hand, we were the first Europeans to take an examination of this kind at such a renowned university in China, and we were repeatedly reminded of this privilege. It was, in short, a great honour. We in our turn acknowledged this in view of the fact that hundreds, if not thousands, of doctors and healers at home practised a mere 'stabbing around' with needles which is called 'acupuncture' in the West without having a professional expert to guide them in Chinese medical matters. In fact, there is not one teacher in Europe who teaches this subject correctly.

In the evening, we listened to 'music' in the room of Aladin Bailey, our colleague from Chad. It was little more than a wild, very loud African rooting and tooting. Aladin, Adnan and Balu found it simply wonderful. Then there followed a sample of Chinese music in European style, to some extent arranged 'communistically'. This did not appeal to either Achille or me.

Further Experience in the Clinic and the University

Yesterday in the clinic we had a few children as patients. One of these, a little girl, was two-and-a-half years old and had bronchitis. We looked at her small tongue, which was red and covered with a thick white coating. She was running a temperature of 38°C. The needles were inserted quite briefly but deeply, and immediately withdrawn again by old Dr Ou-Yang. The child squealed, but then waved goodbye to us, half laughing, half crying.

Apparently, the children learn this kind of thing in kindergarten. Our particular child showed itself as 'revolutionary' in a way in that it was encouraged by its mother, by calling out, 'Dear doctors, dear foreign guests!' The whole thing was quite farcical.

The second child was a baby of two-and-a-half months suffering from some intestinal disturbance. In this case, too, the needles were inserted very quickly, but not deeply, by the old Chinese doctor and immediately withdrawn. The child uttered no protest.

During treatment, other children stood around us and the Chinese kept saying, 'Hao-le, Hao-le,' which means something like: 'It's all right; it'll be all right again soon!' With this they wanted to calm down the children who made a terrible hullabaloo and who were trembling all over while they were treated.

The younger the children were, the fewer cries of pain they uttered. The older ones, on the other hand, cried and shouted on being acupunctured just like children in Europe. Up to now, we had not seen anything spectacular. Patients lay there quite still and waited for 'De-Qi' – that is, for the 'arrival of the Qi' sensation. If this then happened, they did not cry out, but carefully waved a hand, nodded, or quietly gave a vocal signal to the doctor that he could stop further stimulation, which was carried out by either turning the needle or moving it up or down.

Finally, a very pretty young woman arrived for treatment. She was immediately isolated from us westerners and taken to a far corner of the room and treated there in the dark where no one could see her. Neither were we allowed to read her medical report, despite the fact she had been brought to us for treatment. The oldest physician, Dr Ou-Yang, in the meantime applied acupuncture to her separately behind a curtain. We were not permitted to treat this young person because it was feared that our treatment could lead to closer contact, and who could know what sort of consequences that could have! Here, great care was taken in terms of contact between the sexes and every effort was made to avoid any kind of communication between Chinese and Europeans – including medical contact.

In the afternoon at the institute our teachers talked with us about the four diagnostic methods – those of seeing, listening, smelling and touching – as well as the Eight Guiding Principles, Ba Gang, of the so-called differentiation of Chinese diagnoses, Bian-Zheng, which is taught here in a funny imitation of the doctrine of Marxian dialectic materialism, and which is named 'dialectic diagnosis'. Bian-Zheng does not represent a correct translation of the theory and methods of ancient Chinese medicine, but is an attempt to bring these traditional ideas into line with modern party-political thinking. As a consequence, it is useful in a financial and expedient way for such institutions as the Academy for Chinese Medicine in Shanghai to push it into the foreground and let it enjoy pecuniary support.

Below us, we could hear the rhythmical stamping of Chinese worker and farmer students as they recited the Chinese names of acupuncture structures: 'Huan Tiao Yu Yang Ling. He Dan Yong Fa Dan, He Jie Yong Fa Jie, San Bai Liu Shi Xue, Bu Chu Shi Er Jie'.

Gradually, I, too, was falling prey to the impression that I was living in a madhouse.

Some Chinese doctors in this country have succeeded in selling their ancient healing methods as 'revolutionary' to their party bosses and they, in their turn, as a pretty stupid organisation, have not even noticed the dull deviations of these methods from the old Chinese characters.

I sat next to Achille and drew the two different characters for 'diagnosis' into his folder for him. They were 'Bian', 辨, on one side and 'Bian', 辯, on the other. The first one is the term for a medical diagnosis – what we do in the clinic; it is written with 'dao', 刂, 'knife', in its centre; the second one is that for 'dialectic reasoning', and it has 'yan', 言, in the middle. This Bian, 辯, is common to communist theory. In the communist abbreviation – the Maoist form, that is – it is written today as 辩, which, at a glance, can easily be confused with the first character, 辨. However, mixing up things like this displays considerable literary ignorance, something that is quite characteristic of Chinese party circles today. Both of these characters are derived from the old symbol 辡, Bian, which in fact shows two criminals who mutually accuse one another. Moreover, vocalised in the same fourth tone as well, Bian, 辫, means 'to plait'. A 'Bian-zi', 辫子, is a Chinese plait, a pigtail, and confusingly, with exactly the same pronunciation, 'Bian', 便, means 'convenience' or 'human excrement'. 'Da Bian', 大便, is, then, shit and 'Xiao Bian', 小便, is 'urine', 'pee'.

'Has Chinese medicine to do with shit, then?' asked Achille.

'Well, certainly Marxist dialectics has to do with ordure,' I mocked.

'I mean as far as pronunciation goes.'

'Sure.'

'And with the old Chinese plait, too?'

'You have to be able to correctly differentiate between the characters, Achille.'

In the meantime, our Chinese teachers described the methods of tongue diagnostics to us.

Achille again and again shook his head and kept murmuring: 'This here is really the very first plait. It's worse than Hippocrates. Do we as modern doctors have to swallow all this humbug? We know already that a furred tongue is not normal. Why warm it all up for us?'

And he added in French: '*Je ne comprends pas la langue chinoise.*'

This could mean either that he did not understand the Chinese language or that he did not understand the Chinese method of tongue diagnosis.

In the evening we visited a ballet performance with the title *The Society of Dagger Fighters*. This was a group of men in Shanghai who conspired to oppose their white colonial masters in the last century, a theme dear to the hearts of all party members. The white, long-nosed colonialists were portrayed as ridiculous and disagreeable. From the point of view of choreography, the presentation of the British ambassador, a Catholic priest, European soldiers and other high-ranking people in uniform with weapons, for example, was quite amusing. However, as far as these western people were concerned, there was apparently nothing good at all to say about them. The Catholic priest was subjected to particularly contemptuous treatment. The actor crossed himself constantly and held the Bible ostentatiously in front of the noses of the public. Caricatures of western people such as this are continuously being presented to the public in China, so that it is small wonder that antipathy and misunderstanding abound. The whole thing was nothing less than a campaign of hate and contempt. It was here that the reason was to be found for the considerable mistrust against us that was prevalent in a great part of the Chinese population.

ID Card to Swim

We all experienced something insidious when we expressed the desire to swim. It was now the end of May and the weather had become very close in Shanghai. We badly needed to cool down. For this, we were told, we needed a 'paper', and to acquire this we needed to undergo a health test. This, in turn, required that we had our blood tested, had an X-ray and underwent a complete medical check-up at one of the main hospitals. Only when all this had been completed and found to be satisfactory would we receive a special Chinese certificate allowing us to swim in China. Sans ID, no swimming!

'For heaven's sake!' we said. 'We're all of us experienced medical folks and know for sure whether we're healthy or not!'

But that was of no consequence to the Chinese. 'A regulation is a regulation,' they repeated.

'And who's responsible here?' we asked.

'The party, of course!'

'And how about our own self-determination, eh?'

'As western doctors you have no say in these matters here.'

Walo, the Swiss surgeon from Lausanne, asked politely whether each of us had handed in our European 'I' – our individual Ego and our personal being – together with our entry permit on arrival in China, but this was either ignored or not understood at all by the interpreters.

None of our political warders (I could no longer call them political guides) knew what a European 'I' was. They shrugged their shoulders and shook their heads.

Finally, it came down to us being obliged to be examined from head to toe. The doctors in charge of this very important mission were not even in a position to properly carry out such a duty. This was soon quite clear to us all. They tapped at our knees with small rusty hammers, but not at the right place on the patella tendon, and so produced no reaction from us. They wanted of course to test the neural condition within the nervous system, but obviously knew nothing about it. No one had ever clarified the situation to them or shown them how to manage it. They simply went through the motions as though they understood them as well as western medical personnel. A French doctor in our company, Lagarde, the anaesthetist from Paris, wanted to assist and to show them the correct examination procedure. He was rudely bawled at and told to mind his own business. After all, he was the patient, and a foreigner, a Wai-Guo-Ren, to boot.

'Shut up and do what the "doctor" tells you!'

'Doctor? What kind of "doctor" is this?' asked Achille.

While we waited our turn, Achille recounted one of his jokes. He probably thought of it because the examining doctors insisted on being addressed as 'doctor'. At least this was what the interpreters told us.

'They demand this title because the truth is that they aren't really doctors,' Achille said. 'What kind of academic degree have they got, then? An MD, a PhD or a Doctor of Medicine, or something? They merely mistake our western medical degree for their profession. Do you know what happened to me in New York once when I was with a group of African colleagues at a WHO conference there?'

We were curious.

'The Africans, like us, had to sign their immigration forms. For some, this was rather laborious. One of them simply put three crosses at the appropriate place on the form.

' "What's this?" the duty officer enquired with suspicion.

'The black colleague beamed: "The first cross is my family name."

' "And the second?"

' "My forename."

'The American, a little irritated by this, then asked, "And the third?"

'The African smiled angelically and modestly replied, "That means 'Doctor'."'

Adnan, our colleague from Cameroon, now stood up. He laughed uproariously, and slapped Achille's thigh with such a resounding smack that he called out in alarm: 'Ouch!'

'What an ugly story, Achille,' he sang, 'but it could be so, could be so; I know my Africans.'

'Good that Balu and the other Africans are not here; they would have told you a thing or two,' the Swiss, Reto Armbruster, grinned.

But Adnan could take a joke. Only he, we West Europeans, one Syrian and the Persians wanted to go swimming. The other Africans, the Laotians and the Sri Lankans were used to the heat, and our two Dutch ladies had no interest in water derived from Chinese lakes and rivers. 'It will damage our fair Dutch skin,' they feared.

At the door of the waiting room we could hear the doctors and sisters rowing with each other. It was a general fact that doctors here were coarse and authoritarian towards their patients and towards the nurses. We experienced this every day in the clinic.

We, the prospective swimmers, were aware that they wanted to teach us our place, because the party didn't wan't us to swim. Gradually, we became rather irritated by this game. First of all, they made us wait in a dark, stuffy room where we had to entertain ourselves with jokes, and then, after this interval, we were asked in two by two.

Blood was taken without a hitch. Then we were told to appear the next day for an X-ray. We protested at this, since one of the Frenchmen had seen X-ray apparatus in the next room.

'There's the X-ray,' he said, 'we can use that thing.'

'It's probably out of order,' said Achille with sepulchral wisdom.

'No,' said one of the Swiss drily, 'it's worse than that. I've had a glance at the old thing. It was manufactured in Berlin in 1925. You can still read the rusty inscription on the side. In Europe at that time there were no radiation safety measures. This X-ray examination could be a hundred times more risky for us than any kind of swimming. I think we'd better give the idea up.'

Was it possible for us at this stage to object to the whole unreasonable business and also to the real danger we were to be literally exposed to? We would certainly not receive a swimming 'paper' if we did object, yet that was just the thing we wanted as it had become intolerably hot in the last few days. Our daily round of work from Monday through to Saturday was quite demanding. In the morning we had three hours of clinical work with many patients, and in the afternoon, four hours of lectures and practice. In the evening we had to learn what had been taught, and three times a week we had Tai-Ji-Quan on the hotel roof. We just needed to swim to cool off and refresh ourselves.

After endless debate and excited discussion on the part of our Chinese colleagues, we were allowed to stay to be X-rayed. We neither needed to take our clothes off or otherwise to remove parts of our clothing. Each one of us was shoved in front of the frosted-glass panel, followed by an assistant moving a huge lever switch, a whining sound, a clatter and a bang, a large arc of blue and then … 'Next one!'

One of our company who had already had some experience with these instruments that were worthy to go into a museum was of the opinion that the old thing had long since given up the ghost. And Albert, the Frenchman, wanted to see the results.

'We never show them to patients!' one of the Chinese retorted.

Well, good, if that was the case, then there would be no X-rays to look at and no fear either of radiation. Despite that, an X-ray had to be made; that was the order. In this way, the Marxist system and the revolutionary order, as it was called, prevailed. Apparently, everything had to be of the very best.

'Long live the Great Helmsman!' Achille squealed.

'He's been dead some time,' Adnan reminded him.

'But he's still steering – where to, God alone knows!'

Then our Swiss surgeon, Walo, appeared and whispered to us: 'All clear, friends, all clear. The cable is not connected to the supply. It's lying on the floor behind the machine. I just had a quick look around a minute or two ago.'

'But where did the din and the flash come from, then?'

'A typical Chinese placebo effect,' Achille concluded.

We assumed that the party was obliged to enter something at some point about our general state of health. A swimming ID examination was a good excuse. A unique chance indeed to examine a prominent group of foreign doctors from head to toe. And what an opportunity! It was a glorious occasion to document whether their bodies were healthy or had been eaten up by liberal, cabbalistic poison, an opportunity to confirm whether they were suffering from syphilis, athlete's foot, gonorrhoea, hepatitis, cancer, scabies or paranoia. What a windfall for the bloodhounds of the communist secret service.

After this farce, we all had to climb a storey higher, where a bevy of 'five-hole doctors' (the name here for ENT and eye specialists) were waiting to receive us.

Hardly had I entered the room when a woman behind a face mask, a sister (or was she a female doctor?) with an ophthalmoscope on her head, ran after me, grabbed me without any kind of introduction and began to turn my right eyelid up for examination, twisting up the lid to the exterior for investigation. She did not succeed and then brutally pulled at the lid for a second try, so that it became very painful. I had also had a year's specialist training in this area, and had often carried out this examination myself. In the first place, such an examination was completely senseless, since this is only necessary when there happens to be a foreign body in the eye, or in the case of a slipped contact lens, or where there is suspicion of a tumour or a trachoma, which is an African eye disease. None of this was relevant to me in any way. Moreover, the way this woman went about such an examination was so primitive that any European student in his or her clinical term would have made a better job of it.

I roared at her in pain: 'Bu hao! What the devil do you think you're doing?'

Shocked at this, she let go of my eyelid, took a small lamp, and looked tentatively first into the left eye (apparently she encountered nothing here) and then into the right. Then she said that everything was in order. It remained a mystery to me what she saw or what she had wanted to see.

During the whole procedure she trembled and waggled her legs backwards and forwards rhythmically, which I found especially irritating. Many Chinese fidget like this and I find it a particularly annoying habit. They believe this to be a means of reducing weight.

Then a second woman appeared, attired like the other in a white coat, her face covered with a mask, and she held an otoscope in her hand. She thrust the pipe-like instrument so deeply into my auditory opening that she seemed to penetrate through the ear into the skull. She forcibly touched the membranes of the periosteum of my mastoid bone. I cried out in pain. I have done this simple technique, too, many times in my life and have applied it again and again to my patients at home. This woman, active in the specialist department of a Shanghai hospital, clearly had no idea how to carry out the simple examination. Or was it that the anatomical condition of the auditory canal of the Chinese was different from that of the Europeans?

I asked her what she was up to, and again the woman let me go.

A third woman, this time bespectacled but in a similar mask, appeared and wanted to look into our noses, whereupon she prised open our nostrils, one after the other, with the forceps she had with her, so she could inspect what was inside. Her first victim was Adnan, the friendly fat native of Cameroon. He patiently shoved his broad proboscis out for her from which a veritable bush of black hair protruded. The next was the Swiss surgeon, Walo. On this occasion, he insisted on a fresh forceps, if you please, for use on his Helvetian conk. The hairy nostrils of his colleague Adnan were apparently not to his taste. But at this juncture there appeared to be some kind of problem. He was told that in this 'five-hole' university clinic department there was in fact only one pair of forceps for such a job. This pair was used for every patient without any sterilisation in between, since to do so would take all day. We informed her that such a procedure was not possible as it was an infringement of the basic laws of hygiene.

The director of this 'five-hole' establishment had been standing around during these procedures and had smoked one cigarette after another in the clinic room. Now he raised his unpleasant voice to tell us that we would have to appear again next week if we wanted an ID swimming card.

Then I had to take off my shirt and lie down on a couch. I wondered at this, because this place was supposed to be the ENT department, and therefore had nothing to do with internal medicine. A woman, probably a kind of assistant doctor, now aimlessly began to knead my abdomen. It was ridiculous. I asked her in Chinese what organ she had just come across: '"Pi" (spleen), "Gan" (liver), "Wei" (stomach), "Xiao-Chang" (small intestine), "Da-Chang" (large intestine)?' at which she fell into a fit of laughter, so that her hands lost all strength to massage. She gasped for breath and said by way of what was a kind of diversion that I spoke quite good Chinese. Then she did the same as before with my back.

Again I followed her movements with my comments, referring to 'Fei' (lungs), 'Xin' (heart) and 'Shen' (kidneys) – and all this tickled the little doctor to death. From a medical point of view, the whole thing was merely a ritual. At the end of the examination, she declared that everything was 'Hen Hao' – that is, 'very good'. She wrote a few things on her protocol pad. I was discharged and could now put my clothes on again.

Then the department's head pulled out a long spatula, took hold of colleague Haubensack, illuminated his gullet and diagnosed acute tonsillitis.

Achille protested at this. He had felt nothing in his throat to complain about and had had no inflammation of that kind since childhood. The interpreters translated this.

But our Chinese friend remained unimpressed.

'Bian-Tou-Ti Yan', he shouted several times: 'Tonsillitis!'

Achille tapped his forehead and told him he had gone mad. That helped him not at all.

'Benzling!' the Chinese ordered.

'What? Does he want to insult me?' Achille asked. 'I'm not a Benzling – rather, I'm something of a cheeky bastard, a rough diamond perhaps, and sometimes even a darling.'

'Benzling, Benzling!' the Chinaman crowed, at the same time making a movement with his hand as though he were pressing something into his mouth.

One of the sisters (still muffled in her mask) brought a brown jar with white tablets in it.

Achille said to him in French: 'Ta geule! Keep your mouth shut!' But the interpreters refused to translate that.

'Benzling,' the five-hole manager demanded for the umpteenth time.

I took the jar out of the sister's hand and read what was on its label in the smallest print: 'Penicillin'. So that was it!

'By "Benzling", he didn't mean you, dear Achille,' I said. 'He meant "Pe-ni-cil-lin" – here! He can't pronounce it properly, you see. You'll have to take them pills.'

'No thanks,' Achille replied. 'He can take them himself or stuff them up his arse for all I care!'

The interpreters declined to translate, and the Chinese remained resolute.

Achille now drew himself up to his full height, stood squarely before this Chinese, who was already rather unsteady on his legs, and waved his hands close to the man's face, this way and that.

'Hula-hula-hula,' he mimicked, 'you big, big, big medicine man.'

The Chinese doctor put on an embarrassed smile.

'You no doctor, but me doctor,' continued Achille.

In a kidney dish lay a dirty scalpel.

'I now take knife!'

Achille seized the instrument and made designs in the air, one or two professional incisions from which one could easily see that he was a master of his craft.

The interpreters translated all this now as well as they could.

The ENT boss began to tremble. The examination was broken off immediately. We were now told that everything, yea, everything was very good. 'Hen Hao!'

We were all perfectly sound in mind and limb and could leave. Achille's performance had quite overwhelmed this 'five-hole' man. Baring his teeth and in total embarrassment, he put out his hand, twice to one or two of us, probably because he could not tell us apart for sheer excitement. Shaking our heads, we trotted down the stairs, where the bus was waiting for us.

This episode, which had annoyed us all, had highlighted how 'advanced' western medicine in China was. Apparently, one was not in a position here to estimate and apply the relative importance of individual examination methods, techniques that we employ and coordinate every day in Europe. Here, rather, one went through a scheme of medical investigation mechanically, but did not understand what the examination method meant at all. One tapped here or there, then somewhere else, looked here or there and sometimes in another place, pressed here or there or somewhere else.

Exactly that which we were taught yesterday during the course at the academy about how important it was to understand the individual results of an examination in Chinese medicine and so judge the particularity of a patient was totally lacking here in the application of modern western medicine. The people ostentatiously went through the motions of applying their methods, but did not really understand what they were in fact doing. It was merely a sort of pantomime. The reason for this may be that here western medicine is hugely overestimated. On the other hand, it has not been properly processed in China. I feel strongly that some of this inadequacy is due to the extremely short amount of time allowed for the study of western medicine in red China.

It is possible that our Chinese colleagues will say, 'Very well, but you people haven't understood Chinese medicine likewise. You carry out a sort of acupuncture, you use moxa burning methods without having really understood our ancient methods of healing.'

The truth is these are two completely different methods of healing.

Later, at the hotel, I asked Achille whether he was not afraid of the possible consequences of his outburst of anger. Laughing, he shook his head.

'And even if there are consequences,' he said laconically, 'then I'll just go home, that's all. I'm fed up to the teeth with this place anyway.'

We were quiet and drank our red tea.

'No,' Achille continued, 'I have troubles of a quite different nature. I fear that they'll examine us for our sperm count and discover this serious disease in us from which, apparently, many Chinese males suffer – spermatorrhea. If they discover this in us, then we certainly will not be allowed to swim. In such a case we could saturate a whole swimming pool with our capitalistic sperm and all the Chinese virgins coming after us would become pregnant. And that without experiencing the slightest pleasure! The result would be bastards galore, spawned from capitalistic and socialist genetic make-up.'

'We would have by then long since returned to Europe,' he continued, 'but there would be a grave diplomatic crisis between China and the European states and it would be a bad day for Chinese–European friendship. You see, I have a few reservations about this whole business. Just wait and see, Ralf, if they don't take our trousers down to ferret around for this horrible Chinese disease transmitted to us.'

But no one came to take our trousers down. Had Chinese prudery saved the day? Anything which lay below the belt, so to speak, was in any case taboo and was of no interest to anyone here. At least not officially or publicly.

After two days we received our swim card furnished with a passport picture which we, incidentally, had to have made. This quasi ID card had one useful side effect: we were now registered as official members of a unit called the 'University College of Chinese Medicine' in Shanghai, and with this 'paper' we were officially recognised and confirmed. The strange thing was, however, that I was the only one in the group who finally went swimming, because there was no longer any opportunity to swim. The party had made it impossible. On the other hand, the small card did us good service; it was a kind of official key, but more about this later.

Chinese and Western Surgery

One evening there was a knock on the door just as we were preparing our study. It was Lao Lu, our organisation manager, with two of the interpreters. They hardly waited to be asked in and were suddenly in the middle of our room. There was always someone knocking on the door with a letter or just wanting to say something unimportant. There was hardly a moment for reflection. Visitors never came straight to the point. We were always first asked whether the food was acceptable, whether we felt well, and whether we slept well. What did this man want? we asked ourselves. There was a prelude as usual, and we were first asked how the Tai-Ji-Quan was coming along and whether we had mastered its techniques … I got straight to the point:

'Excuse me, but what do you want just at this time?'

The accompanying interpreter was clearly embarrassed. He translated my rather direct enquiry, and old Lu was quick to respond. It concerned our three surgeons who wanted permission after the course to stay on for some weeks and accompany the famous Dr Chen in Hospital No. 6 during his transplantation work. We had been visiting Dr Chen and his hospital and Achille had been impressed by their surgical techniques, which were absolutely western style. Lu looked serious and told us that this was a very difficult matter to arrange. It could only be arranged, he said, in cooperation with the respective governments in Beijing, Switzerland, Germany and France. The reason for this was that one did not know whether such additional information was acceptable to the individual European governments.

Achille went red in the face. Angrily, he asked, 'What's that to do with my government? I'm a citizen of a democratic state, and my state's welfare depends on its taxpayers and electorate and finally, I, Achille Haubensack, am, in the last analysis, the law-maker of this state. Above all, I am a free European and decide on these matters myself. My government doesn't give a damn!'

'Well, things are different here,' Lu replied patiently. 'As our guests, you should know this by now.'

We happened to be here in China, he said, and for that reason had to abide by its regulations. We had received permission to come here and study acupuncture. But nothing more.

'You can go to the devil with your bloody acupuncture,' Achille said. 'It's all a lot of humbug and you can be sure that we'll report on it when we get back to Europe.'

'Oh,' Lu said in a small voice, 'please don't do that.'

'Oh yes, we'll do so,' Achille countered. 'I'm wasting my precious time here, playing about with all this medical eyewash. I want to see something for all this nonsense – if there's anything in it at all – so that we can profit from the knowledge at home. So far, I can see nothing of value in this wretched country.'

The old man kept his fists on the flag. We had received exceptional permission to study acupuncture. If this permission were now to be changed to include the wish to study transplantation surgery, then there would have to be prior diplomatic negotiation between the states concerned, and it was not certain whether our states would allow such an extended course of study.

'Did you ask our respective states whether we could go swimming or not?' Achille asked sarcastically.

Lu was now visibly uncomfortable. 'No, we have made no such application.'

'You see,' Achille pursued, 'it could well have been that our governments were not in agreement with our wish to swim. What then, eh? A very serious political crisis would have been the consequence.'

Lu looked numbed. His face was suddenly a visage carved from criss-crossed furrows.

'There'll be a political scandal, mon cher Monsieur Lu,' Achille added scornfully.

'That was undertaken by our party as an exceptional case and at its own risk,' Lu stammered.

'Did you ask our governments in Europe or at least their respective representatives in Beijing whether your doctors were allowed to take samples of our blood? It could well be that our governments were not at all in favour of that kind of thing.'

Lu became more and more uncomfortable. 'Why should that be?' he asked.

'Why? Because your apparatus and equipment is completely out of date,' Achille replied.

'How do you know that?' Lu asked, astonished.

Achille laughed. 'Because you can see it engraved on your old stuff:

"Manufactured in Berlin, 1925". That thing's a public danger. In my hospital, where I happen to be the boss, the police would be the first on the scene and then the public prosecutor if someone reported the matter.'

Lu retrieved his composure and countered: 'The equipment we have is safe enough. If it's safe for China, then it is for the rest of the world.'

The interpreter either could not or would not translate this. Large pearls of sweat had stood on his forehead for some time. Suddenly, he was no longer able to interpret. Exhausted, he sank into an armchair and talked about food to divert the course of the conversation.

'Are you satisfied with your food?'

Achille shook his head. 'No. But it's good enough for us.'

Lu then asked whether we were interested in a trip to a community in the country. The conversation stumbled on for another half hour until it was about ten o'clock. Lu then said that we were all probably very tired and we said our goodbyes. Soon after, the Swiss surgeon came by to discuss the Chinese rejecting our wishes. It was well after midnight before we got to bed.

On the following evening I wanted to catch up on the previous evening's loss of time, but I had hardly sat down at my desk when there was another knock on the door and yesterday's two spectres of gloom were standing there again. They were grinning and swayed from one foot to the other.

'No,' I said, 'it really is inconvenient this time. We must do some homework in order to be ready for the course tomorrow.'

Their grins broadened. 'Fu-shi, fu-shi,' the interpreters paraphrased my words. This means, 'Recapitulation of material to be learned'. They said that they would come back later. At ten thirty there was another knock on the door. Achille was already asleep in bed, and had been snoring like a walrus for a good half hour.

'We would like to speak to Monsieur Haubensack.'

I replied, 'Come in, please, and see for yourself. He's been in bed for an hour.'

'Oh, il dormi ... he's asleep! Then we'll do it tomorrow.'

We agreed on this. I drew the interpreters' attention in passing to the fact that the phrase was not 'il dormi', but 'il dort', but they seemed not to be interested. Both merely laughed uneasily and said that I was only a German and for this reason could not know anything of what was correct in French.

We had very little personal freedom and practically no privacy, which was worse. I was glad that the lectures had been cancelled for the day. This would help me to catch up with my work, which had been unwillingly neglected. So I practised Tai-Ji for half an hour. The teacher found for us was friendly and cultured. For him it was clear that we found it difficult to deal with the revolutionary atmosphere in this country. Here, it was the masses, the proletariat and the roughnecks who were the order of the day. People with their own ideas, capabilities and inclinations or those with what we in the West call good manners were all outsiders.

We noticed that this was the case with Dr Chen, the surgeon-in-chief of Shanghai Hospital No. 6. He was not able even to respond to an invitation to Europe in the interests of medical science made by one of our group. He bowed stiffly and silently several times, but was unable to say anything before having talked to the appropriate revolutionary body. Finally, he said: 'I'm sorry, but you will have to consult the health ministry in Beijing about that.'

In addition, Dr Chen was a chain smoker and lit up one cigarette after another. It was certainly possible that he was suffering from severe emotional tension, despite the fact that he was a member of the Shanghai City Revolutionary Committee and, on top of this, a world-famous surgeon. It certainly was not easy for him to live comfortably in this political atmosphere.

Progress in Tai-Ji-Quan

To return to Tai-Ji-Quan for a moment, these exercises were pretty demanding from the point of view of requiring considerable concentration. After a strenuous day in the clinic and with the evenings needing study, Tai-Ji exercises on top of this made for a rather full day. However, these exercises created a feeling of relaxation and freshness. Concentration on the exercises produced a revitalisation of the organism as a whole. This feeling, I believe, was really the result of these regenerative postures. We did them outside on the balcony of the hotel, and if it rained, inside. Sometimes we went downstairs to practise in the parking area behind the hotel. Yesterday we practised in the large hotel foyer in front of a hairdresser's. There were always Chinese spectators. Some of them even joined our group and participated. They probably did this because our teacher was a very good one. He was able to demonstrate the individual exercises with masterly competence. The gatecrashers profited, too, from his presence.

The group of participants was growing. It had got round that the practice was very beneficial. The tall, fat African, Adnan, who had at first laughed at us, joined in yesterday and practised with us very seriously. But his movements were too large and too wild, and he found difficulty in imitating the graceful swinging movements of the Chinese master. Adnan's clumsiness looked dreadfully grotesque, but it made him very happy nevertheless. We

Europeans, I as a German, and the Swiss and the French folks, gave the impression of being gnarled and inflexible. Erazay from Bordeaux, a typical intellectual, first dissected each exercise into its component parts, wanted to know ten times what each individual partial exercise meant and then tried to put everything together. This produced the effect of 'woodenness', rather like a living gearwheel that, when it turns, grinds. Our teacher, however, made all the movements appear as though they arose and ended in one process.

Again, I had just sat down to work when there was a knock on the door. I informed Lu and his interpreter that I had to work and did not wish to be disturbed. They came in nevertheless and each sat down, uninvited, in a chair. I took my paper, my pencil and my books, and withdrew to a corner. Seeing this, the interpreter began to speak in a loud voice, so that I felt particularly disturbed. We Europeans have quite a different method of learning compared with the Chinese. We concentrate intensely and so learn with a high degree of effectiveness.

Loud Music, the Street Committee and a Snooper

After lunch I wanted to take a nap, but just at this moment there was a sudden noise in front of my door coming from a loudspeaker. Revolutionary songs filled the air. I went outside and asked them to stop. The room boys were flabbergasted at this. That was beautiful music, they said, and although we Europeans had good taste in these matters, we didn't have taste and understanding for China's culture and art. Nevertheless, they turned the music off, and this was probably an act of politeness towards the guest. If I had been Chinese, the noise would have gone on unabated. No Chinese here has a right to a private life – not even in his own four walls is he allowed to do what he likes. The folks from the 'street committee' come along to check on everything and it is they who determine what he or she does in the apartment and what he or she may have in it, what pictures may hang on the walls – and of course a picture of the 'Great Helmsman' must be omnipresent. They also determine what books are on the shelves, and as well as no one having a right to private life, no one can desire something for himself or possess something for himself. Even the bedroom is controlled by such committees.

Again I was strongly reminded of the Nazi terror in Germany. On one day in spring 1942 the doorbell rang at our place at about six in the evening.

A huge, broad-shouldered man in SA uniform stood there and demanded entry. He stepped into the house without being formally asked to do so.

He removed his officer's cap with its highly polished peak and introduced himself as 'Peymann'. I remember my younger brother saying, 'Uncle Peymann, are you a "Polizei-Mann" (a policeman)?' That is just what he looked like and my brother was pleased, because, for him, policemen were something to be admired and, after all, the words rhymed well.

'No, my young German hero,' said the broad-shouldered fellow, shoving his gnarled, chewing muscles forward, together with his massive jawbone. He thrust out his brutal chin: 'I'm a Partei-Mann (a party man).' That rhymed, too, which pleased my brother so much that he started to jump up and down.

'That's it, now. I have come to you from the party,' the officer announced to my frightened mother, who did not defend herself against this intruder as he began to open doors and make himself present in other rooms. He picked up newspapers and thumbed through them and then turned to the bookshelves in the lounge. My father was at the front and so there was nothing to hinder this creature from doing what he liked on our premises.

'What party do you belong to, then?' my mother asked shyly.

'There's only one party and you should know that,' he replied to my browbeaten mother, looking at her accusingly. 'Only one for our Fatherland, and that's the N-S-D-A-P.' He spelled out the letters like a machine. 'That's what you have to tell your children every day. You have to ask them these five holy letters, so that they can quickly learn them for good and never forget them: ENN-ESS-DEE-A-PEE!'

I well remember that he coughed these individual letters rather than spelled them out, with the result that he hissed between the black gaps of his teeth and sent out spittle through them in our direction, so that we had to wipe our faces. My two brothers thought this was delightfully funny and laughed at the outrage.

My mother summoned the last of her courage. 'What do you want here?' she enquired.

'I have the job of making sure whether the right National Socialist tone is to be found in your house,' he blustered.

This he uttered curtly like an order. He was, so to speak, the 'street committee' in person.

'Excuse me,' said my mother, 'my children are three, six and nine years of age and my husband is at the front, what other convictions could we have than the real German ones?'

'That's by no means so sure,' said Peymann and walked towards the open piano.

'Now there we are! What do I see on the music stand: *Songs without Words.* First of all, there are no songs without words, because all songs have words. That's why they are songs! You've only to think of the magnificent party songs, the lieder of the ENN-ESS-DEE-A-PEE'.

He spat the words again and again we children laughed. Peymann, though, didn't allow himself to be put off by this.

'For example: "Es zittern die morschen Knochen" [The brittle bones are trembling]. Now there's a song for you! And to match it, an immortal, wonderful melody on top! That's what you should play and sing to your children every day, Frau er, er ...'

'Can you sing it for us, Uncle?' my little brother asked. Herr Peymann cleared his throat several times and indeed was about to sing this Nazi ditty, but then thought better of it, and turned to more important matters.

'And who composed these "songs without words", do you know? Frau er ... er? I'll tell you. It was a certain Felix Mendelssohn, a Jew, the son of Mendel, as the name suggests. That doesn't belong in a German household, and certainly not one with children. I could of course confisiate [he probably meant "confiscate"] this music, but this time I'll leave it to you to destroy it. You'll place it in the waste-paper basket, do you understand?'

'But it's lovely music,' my mother complained in subdued tones.

Herr Peymann stamped his cloven foot in protest, both feet enclosed in most highly polished boots.

'An outrage, that's what it is!' he shouted. 'Frau So-and-So! An outrage. This miserable piece of Jew-crap. The muck goes into the waste-paper basket, do you understand!?'

Now he turned to the writing desk. On it stood a picture of my father in army uniform.

'Aha, der Papa, but where is a picture of our leader, Adolf Hitler, Frau er ... er, where? Show it to me!'

'We have no such picture,' said my mother.

'Sooo, Frau er, er ... No Hitler picture in the house, but on the other hand, a piece of perverse Jew-music on the piano. Is that your genuine German attitude, eh?'

My little brother had run into the neighbouring room and returned with a picture. He collected cigarette pictures, which he placed in a large album.

'I've a picture here of Ardoof Flitscher,' he said triumphantly and shoved the collector's object under the snooper's nose.'

Peymann was impressed.

'Well done, my lad!' he proclaimed. 'You've saved the reputation of the whole family. It's clear that you're going to be a good party member one day. But you can't yet say the name properly. Dreadful! Completely wrong! He's not called "Ardoof", but "Aa-dolllfff". That's a noble name. That is party nobility. You've only got to get the "ell" right, do you understand? And above all, the second part is not "doof", but "DOLF".'

In pronouncing the 'f' of 'doof' [the word 'doof' in German can be compared with 'daft' in English], he spat at us again and we had once again to wipe our faces. 'The tongue must rrrolll!'

'But Ralf is doof,' said the small collector and jabbed me in the side.

Herr Peymann overlooked the incident. 'Hitt-lerr-lerr,' he recited.

My brother echoed this: 'Lerr, lerr, lerr!' He was enjoying himself.

'The lad is only three, Herr Parteimann, er . . . Herr, excuse me, Peymann,' my mother expostulated. 'He can't pronounce everything correctly at this age. That's how it is.'

'And it's exactly for that reason that you will have to practise it with him every day,' said the snooper, pulling himself to his full height. 'I'll come again next week and I want to see a large Hitler picture here, and I don't want to see or hear any "songs without words", do you understand?'

He then fumbled in his pockets and produced a list, turned to the bookcase along the wall and thumbed along the backs of the books. He repeatedly consulted the contents of his booklist, murmured some names, then fished one of the books out and his face went dark. Threateningly, he bawled, 'What have we got here? Heinrich Mann, *Der Untertan*,' and again he looked into his list and related what he had read in it. He continued: '"A book like this, decadent and ruinous for our people, a book which drags the German soul through the muck. Jewish poison!" And that belongs to your household, Frau er . . . er, eh?'

'What you maintain is not correct,' my mother said bravely. 'Heinrich Mann isn't a Jew and neither is his brother Thomas. They are both north German Hansa folks and they have written very amusing books, full of humour and wit. We like reading this.'

'The very name "Mann" shows that he's of Jewish origin,' the nosy parker sniffed arrogantly. 'A real German man is not called "Mann". He IS a man! I can't leave this book here. I will have to confisiate it. Your three boys could be infected by it. It's for your own security, Frau er, er . . . I'll take it with me. Next Sunday at the cemetery behind the church there will be a ceremonial public burning of poisonous rubbish like this. The Führer insists upon it! Heil Hitler!'

'Can we come and see it?' my little brother enquired.

'You are required to be there, my lad. All of you! The blazing fire is your purification. It will be an occasion for celebration too. The Gauleiter from Weser-Ems, Herr Röver, will be there in person. Heil Hitler!'

He stuck out his right arm in salute. Then, the offending book under his left arm, he marched out in goose-step towards the door. There, he placed his cap upon his head, turned to us once more and roared: 'Heil Hitler! Frau er, er . . . Heil Hitler, my lads!'

He came again several times. In the meantime, my mother had procured a picture of our 'Führer' and hung it on the wall of the living room. The Mendelssohn music was banned to the loft. When my father returned on leave in the summer of that year, he showed the brown ruffian the door. He never returned.

This kind of state-instituted slavery – there's no other word for it – is the very worst thing demanded from the Chinese and it is quite similar to the attitude of the Nazi party during its control of German citizens in the early '40s. The state and the party determine what people should read and what kind of music they are permitted to like, what schoolchildren may attend and what profession they may one day exercise. I have often heard that even small children commit suicide in mainland China because they see no dignified way out of this situation. At universities where one expects young people to develop a healthy critical spirit, self-murder among students is unusually high. After all, what are they offered in life? If they are lucky, they receive enough to eat, but that's all. There is no one who can follow his own path.

And when the 'masses' decide that loud music is now to be played, the individual must eat humble pie, just because he is an individual, a creature without rights. And when one comes to think of it, the individual of European tradition, the free citizen, is precisely the conveyor of knowledge, culture and civilisation. There is no such possibility for the collective, the blind masses. It is a pure, reflexive group phenomenon, a mediocrity that can say nothing of the individual human mosaic of which it is made. The occidental philosophical basic view of life is here transformed into its opposite counterpart, and expresses itself as a dominant Chinese social order which is becoming more and more distinct.

As a result of the need to order the masses by the state, there is a tendency, too, with us in the West to increasingly adopt impersonal 'non-values' as a yardstick in our activities. Current western scientific endeavour, represented by our universities and research institutes, shows an alarming tendency to be moving in this direction. Orthodox western medicine is becoming more and more anonymous, for example, but anyone returning from Maoist China will quickly be cured of the desire to criticise what goes on in Europe. He or she returns as a convinced European, and that in the best traditions of occidental thinking.

Today, some Chinese TV reporters appeared again on the scene at the clinic in order to film us as western doctors in the work of administering Chinese acupuncture. We were to be represented in public as well-established western doctors who had come to learn and practise in China what was not available in the West – that is, Chinese needle therapy and moxibustion. This served the propaganda machine very well.

The same TV people were recently in the university to film how we learned and how we studied. I had never seen the Lung-Hua Hospital so thoroughly clean, ordered and decorated as it was on those days on which the TV teams appeared. It was all show. As for us, we had to be filmed taking patients' pulses, making tongue diagnoses and exploring their medical history.

After this, our pre-arranged needle and moxibustion skills were shown.

Achille and I now thought we knew why there were no mentally ill people in the People's Republic of China. The reason was that everyone here was more or less mentally handicapped. The dispensation here was, so to speak, a state-prescribed psychosis maintained by violence, and one which every Chinese man and woman had to be diagnosed with and be told that the situation they suffered from was the norm. When everyone is daubed with the same brush of lunacy, then that is the norm! There were, then, no exceptions, since everyone here had some kind of psychological problem.

Poor Chinese School Education

Yesterday, we had an outing to a so-called middle school, the last educational stage prior to going to university. There was nothing there to see of educational performance, and it was clear that nothing of the sort was required from those attending the school. It was dominated by stupid praise for 'Our Great Chairman' and the Communist Party. Seventeen- to nineteen-year-olds were busy making small pieces of apparatus such as lamps and cycle stands. They were also copying drawings which their teachers had previously set up for them. They sat there, all of them, with their pencils held at the same angle. In the physics lesson, they were looking up at metal balls hanging from the ceiling, and shortly before our visit, mathematical formulae were hurriedly written on the board. One was given the impression that the young people were busy studying these. However, we soon noticed that no one understood anything about physics and mathematics, not even the teacher!

The only foreign language the students knew anything about was English, and this was well below the western average considering their age. Everything gave the impression of being rigged and artificial, there simply to impress visitors. None of them showed any creativity, none of them was eager to discuss anything with us, and their expressions were tired and apathetic. Many of them also appeared to be unwell, their faces pale and anaemic.

The pupils were well below the intellectual level of their western counterparts. Depressed, they sat there, talked endlessly about the Chinese communist revolution, poured tea for themselves and with dead eyes waved Mao's 'Little Red Book' in the air. The whole thing seemed hopeless. Bored, I took up one of these Mao bibles belonging to one of the pupils and looked inside. To my astonishment, I discovered comic illustrations, little frog-eyed Chinese ghosts which, according to the Law of Contradiction, yelled at each other and attacked each other with archaic weapons. There were long-tailed, fire-spitting dragons and bearded wizards flying through the air on what looked like broomsticks. Apparently, it was a special issue for those who could no longer abide the arid words of the 'Great Chairman'. The lad was shocked at my finding the book and tore it out of my hand. I behaved as though I'd not found anything special about it.

In contrast, the small children in the kindergarten still displayed genuine happiness and spontaneity. They laughed and frolicked free from care, because they did not know what was ahead of them in life. These younger children were still intact. They painted pictures that informed and transmitted ideas, and they could set up cheerful little scenes for themselves like all children. In contrast to them, the children of the middle schools seemed to have lost all hope of a life of dignity and humanity.

Today, we spoke of the phenomenon of thriftiness among the Chinese. They throw nothing away, and everything is mended a hundred times if necessary. They appeared in the clinic, for example, in trousers and socks that consisted of one patch over another. There was hardly anything left of the original fabric; the garment was merely a farrago of stitchwork. No one, it seemed, could bring himself to throw old things away. We doctors were of the opinion that it was the same with their old-fashioned medicine. The fact was that the healing traditions still surviving were actually obsolete, and yet no one would throw them overboard and so replace them with more modern methods out of sheer tightfistedness. Rather, their old tradition was patched and added to by western medicine, here a bit and there a bit, in order to give a good impression of progress, but, like their old socks, it was high time it was thrown away and replaced with something more modern and more effective.

VI

We Want to Study Needle Analgesia

Within the framework of our course, we wanted to be instructed in the techniques of acupuncture analgesia. Actually, that was the reason why the anaesthetists among us came here. We had announced this desire on our arrival two months previously, but the academy and the Revolutionary Committee had so far flatly refused to oblige. As a consequence, we had contacted our respective embassies in Beijing in the meantime. Apparently, we were concerned here with 'state secrets', secrets which could not be 'betrayed' to the West. On the other hand, of course, it could also be that needle anaesthesia was still somewhat in its infancy. We could, of course, as experts in our own specialised medical areas, be in a position to 'look into the cards' as it were and so discover the weak points of the method.

Somewhat annoyed, Achille and I talked about the situation of dentistry as we found it here in China. It found itself in a serious dilemma, since no one was allowed to open their mouth. Achille was outraged about it. He said that teeth here had to be pulled through the entire length of the intestinal tract and out through the anus. Here, opening the mouth too wide was a punishable offence carrying heavy penalties. For this reason, aspiring dentists in China were obliged to undergo several semesters of a course in proctology before being allowed to practise tooth extraction. In this, we, as western democrats, were in a much more congenial position, and especially at that present moment since our common advance into the health ministry here in China, for which we hoped for support from our diplomatic representatives. After all, we had been chosen by our own health ministries, placed under diplomatic immunity and sent to China to study acupuncture and analgesia. We noticed what a pleasure it was for us as free people to be able to open our mouths, and we did just that to make our needs clear. However, people here were not used to this. They broke down and then crept off to their respective authorities and kept their own mouths tightly closed. Nevertheless, it was only with determination that anything could be done here. The Chinese could not do this, because the first and most important thing for them to do was to keep their mouths shut and remain silent.

The day before yesterday, we officially informed our Chinese colleagues, the professors, the interpreters and the Revolutionary Committee that our doctors' group would leave as one should the lessons in needle analgesia – that is, surgical operations using acupuncture to kill pain – be withheld from us. Moreover, we would hold a press conference in Paris and tell the world what a miserable state Chinese medicine is in and that we had all returned very disappointed and frustrated. Further, the whole business of acupuncture in our opinion was an unprecedented bluff, a false pretence and pure show designed to bring China into the international foreign policy arena. We were completely in accord with one another and to this end would sign a written resolution to this effect that evening, a copy of which would be sent to our respective embassies in Beijing.

Yesterday went off very quietly. Apparently the Chinese were discussing things behind locked doors. We heard that the university representatives were busy telephoning the health ministry in Beijing. Then, early today, something happened that cheered us all: we were to see an operation conducted under needle anaesthesia for the first time. It concerned the removal of an adenoma of the thyroid under electrically stimulated needle anaesthesia.

It took place in the Lung-Hua Hospital. The patient in this case was an elderly woman of 72 with slightly bluish lips – in other words, suffering from heart insufficiency. She was given two needle insertions on the right and left side of the neck at the points Fu-Tu, and the needles were doubled, should there not otherwise be sufficient mini-volt electricity. Plastic protection had been placed over the needles. An electrical impulse was then led to the needles via a relatively small stimulator. This was enough to produce anaesthesia and the operation could begin. The patient lay for the one-and-half hours of the operation quietly on the operating table and, as she later told us, felt perfectly comfortable. We were all dressed in sterilised clothing, wore protective masks and were even allowed to take photographs.

The anaesthesia and the course of the operation took place as follows:

After two anaesthetists in white coats had introduced the electrical stimulation of the two foramina (points), which took about fifteen minutes, the surgeon, wearing a white head cover, made his appearance. We could see grey hair stubble sprouting from his neck. He nodded to us briefly, then worked quickly and deftly, using a pincette and scalpel. He checked sensitivity to pain at the anterior part of the neck where he was to operate. The patient lay on her back, her head bent a little to the rear.

Achille, who was standing next to me, whispered, 'This approach was first carried out by the Swiss surgeon Emil Theodor Kocher in 1883 – it made him world famous. In 1909, he received the Nobel Prize in Physiology or Medicine. The Chinese have minutely copied his technique.'

The surgeon then opened the skin two centimetres above the jugular notch at the neck and then proceeded to open the skin further, revealing superficial veins from which there was light bleeding. These he capped and went on to enlarge the incision with two hooks placed above and below. Deeper veins were now visible. These, too, were capped and separated. Then the neck facia was split. The neck muscles were loosened from the thyroid gland. There was hardly any blood. The patient could be heard breathing.

The surgeon then asked the patient whether she had any pain. Looking directly into the bright OP lamp above her and shaking her head very slowly, the woman replied, 'Bu tong' – 'no pain'.

The breastbone muscle connecting the larynx and the breastbone and the thyroid muscle were severed in order to gain better access to the thyroid itself.

Beneath, one could see the middle thyroid vein. This was bound twice and severed. One could also see the upper and lower thyroid arteries pulsating. Both of them were bound and cut. Now the thyroid itself could be seen clearly. In the background one could see the aorta beating, as well as the common carotid artery, from which the thyroid artery issues. In front of this the recurrent nerve could be seen crossing it, and it was this that had to be treated with care in order that, after the operation, there would be no damage to the vocal cords that could lead to hoarseness or loss of voice. The right thyroid artery was bound at a reasonable distance from the gland itself in order to protect this sensitive vessel. There was astonishingly little blood loss.

I glanced at the anaesthetist's files. The pulse and the systolic and diastolic blood pressure were running as almost undisturbed horizontal lines, which meant that the patient's blood circulation was in a stable situation. The patient was comfortable, the blinking of her eyes was regular and she breathed rhythmically.

There was a mass of blood vessels in front of the air pipe – the venous arch of the jugulum. All the veins around then were ligatured. Slowly and carefully, all the blood vessels, one by one, were ligatured and severed. The small connection from the air pipe between the two halves of the thyroid was secured by two Kocher clamps. Then it was cut. The larger part of the left side of the thyroid tissue revealed a growth the size of a hen's egg. After the surgeon had clamped the pulsating artery, he removed this lump with scissors. It fell into a kidney dish held for its reception, where it floated in its own serum.

What followed was surgical routine. On both sides of the gland the capsule, left and right, was kept entire. The bean-sized parathyroid glands, which are important for calcium and phosphorous metabolism, were treated carefully. The surgeon then discovered in the tissue to the right of the thyroid another pea-sized growth, which he had not suspected. This he removed. He then proceeded to sew up the gland capsule on the right and left and was once again careful not to damage the recurrent nerve. The neck muscles were once more closed. A drainage tube to collect any blood that might flow from the wound was sewn into the muscle. The facia and the epidermis were sewn together with fine catgut. For cosmetic reasons, the skin of the neck was sewn together by piercing it at regular intervals and using these for the stitches.

'Good work!' said Achille.

The instruments were taken away for sterilisation, the area was cleaned, and the surgeon stood with his hands raised at the end of the operating table.

'How are you feeling?' he asked the patient.

'Hen Hao' – 'very good' – she replied clearly. Now she could get up. Two sisters helped her from the table. For a moment she remained still, having put her feet to the ground. Then she placed her left foot forward and went very slowly towards the door. Once there, she turned and smiled at us, raising her left hand, 'Hsieh-hsieh nimen,' she said. 'Many thanks to you!'

She would remain in the clinic under observation for another couple of days until the drainage application was removed. Then she could return home.

We were impressed. Adnan said, 'The surgeon removed the growths very elegantly. That's fine, but now is the critical time, the actual healing process, and that the woman has to do all by herself. The capacity to heal is the patient's biggest ally, not only for the surgeon, but that goes for all doctors, too. That's the potential, too, from which we create successful acupuncture, and that's what modern western physicians should more clearly realise.'

In Africa, there still seemed to be traces of what once was referred to as 'medical common sense'.

During the drive back, Achille confided to me that 'the real reason why they don't want us to know about their analgesia techniques is that we can then see how minutely they have copied our western surgical techniques as a whole. What we saw today was pure western surgical technique at work. If you take that away, there's not much left over which is of pure Chinese origin! They don't want us to know how carefully they have aped us and then allow us to tell the world about it. And, on the other hand, they certainly don't want us to know how miserably they operate on other occasions.'

'Well, we might perhaps still experience that,' I answered.

'I'm sure we will,' said Achille.

On this occasion, it was clear that the surgeon and his team were of quite another calibre than those encountered in the College of Traditional Chinese Medicine. They were educated and astute people. The surgeon himself spoke comprehensible English and greeted us guests with a nod before addressing himself to the job, later shaking us individually by the hand in farewell. The whole business had style, whereas the traditional teachers who had come with us merely stood around looking a trifle embarrassed. Now and again they tried to tell us something or other, but the attempt in this framework looked rather amateurish. They themselves apparently understand very little about needle analgesia and nothing at all about modern surgery. For my part, I noticed that this patient's pulse and blood pressure had remained astonishingly constant during the whole procedure. Unfortunately, I was not allowed to take a photograph of the anaesthetist's files recording these facts.

After the operation, we were permitted to visit the whole clinic. First of all, we went to the department of traditional Chinese medicine, and then we visited the eye department, ENT and the dental department. We also saw the department for physical therapy, where radiation and electrical stimulation treatment took place. In the dermatological department we came across a piece of laser apparatus put together by the technicians working there, and at the same time we had the opportunity to talk to them about the medical effectiveness of the machine. Here, I had opportunity to speak of my own experience with a laser and described to them the apparatus I worked with in Germany.

Back at our own clinic, we found it was not so full as usual, so that we did not feel as harassed as we did on most days. This left time for discussion. One patient had high blood pressure after having suffered a stroke, and we were afforded the chance to talk about the six different causes of this condition according to Chinese medicine. Today, there was more sun and it was consequently brighter, and this allowed me to take a few photos of my patients.

Just Off to On-Duty Service in Xi-De?

The telephone rang one evening and my wife was on the other end complaining that I was creating problems from faraway China.

'What's happened?' I asked.

'You have your emergency duty call on Wednesday next,' she replied. 'The medical authorities have been ringing every day for a week. If you don't appear for duty, you'll risk a court hearing for failure to render assistance in an emergency.'

'Isn't there anybody else who could take this responsibility?' I enquired. 'There are enough young colleagues who would only be too glad to take this over, because they are just in the process of building up their practices.'

'No. They want you specifically, because you had been delegated three months ago for the job and had flown to China without their consent.'

'And they expect me to fly from China halfway round the world to do duty from Wednesday evening to Thursday early morning and then fly back to China? That's idiotic!'

I immediately thought of Mr Pigface and his wine-reddened nose. Was he doing this to let me know how strong he and his medical henchmen were? One thing was true in all this, and that was that I had left for Shanghai without their permission.

'Do come back, Ralf, otherwise you're in for trouble when you return. They've even threatened to close your practice.'

What should I do? I talked about the matter with Achille.

'They're not so pig-headed as that in France,' he said. 'My colleagues congratulated me on my trip to China, and I managed to find someone to stand in for me immediately. Looks like a relic of your damned Prussian forefathers.' He quoted the German ethics of this time: ' "Üb' immer Treu und Redlichkeit bis an Dein kühles Grab! ['Be honest and true unto thy cool grave']." And it's this grave that your colleagues want to dig for you. Ask your diplomat in Beijing to help you; perhaps he's got a good idea.'

The next morning I rang Beijing. After a minute or two, the ambassador himself was on the other end of the line. He listened to my problem and then simply laughed. He kept on laughing, so that I began to wonder whether he had any understanding for my situation at all. It was embarrassing.

'I'm afraid I can't help you there, Dr Rompard; you'll have to regulate that matter yourself,' he said. 'It has nothing to do with our diplomatic obligations, you see, and I'm sure you understand. However . . .' There was a short pause. 'You'll be receiving a phone call shortly.'

'From whom?'

'I'm not at liberty to say, but not from me, you understand. Please attend very carefully to its contents!'

The bus that was to take us to the university was already waiting. I asked old Mr Lu if I could cycle there later as I didn't want to miss this mysterious message that I was due to receive. I sat in my apartment and waited.

After about a quarter of an hour, the telephone rang. A powerful voice said in English: 'Good morning, Doctor. I have a private and confidential message for you. Please take a piece of paper and write down the following text: "I am ready to fly to Frankfurt next Monday to undertake emergency services on the following Wednesday/Thursday. Please guarantee a first-class Lufthansa return ticket from Shanghai to Frankfurt immediately." End of text. Send this cable to those responsible in Germany immediately. Good luck!'

The conversation had no sooner begun than it ended. Who was the speaker? He had not mentioned a name, and I could not ask, as the phone was instantly hung up. Was the ambassador part of it? I began to reflect. A first-class Lufthansa ticket from Shanghai and back would cost about 8,000 euros. Would the duty organisation over there be prepared to pay out so much for my flight? Never on your life! It was far too niggardly for that kind of thing. Yes, this was the most elegant solution to my problem. I declared my readiness to be there, but insisted at the same time on unacceptable conditions. I was out of the noose. On the way to the university I cycled by the post office and so sent off my telegram using the text recommended to me.

The duty organisation fired back the following morning: 'Suspension of duty while in China.' The secretary had signed the thing

As usual, I went with my colleagues to Hua-Dong Hospital later and did the next treatments there in a much better mood.

A Discussion on the Medical Classics

Afterwards I took a taxi back with Dr Kang and we got out at Fu-Zhou-Lu Street. We went into the antique bookshop, where I managed to find a fine example of the *Huang-Di Nei-Jing Su-Wen*, which had red punctuation in the text and good commentaries. It was brought out in the year 1852 in Soochow. I bought it straightaway. I now possess several editions of this important work, all containing the original version of the text.

We walked down The Bund together in the direction of our hotel. On the way, I asked Kang what it was like in Shanghai before its 'liberation' by the so-called Red Army. He told me that it was pretty bad. The Japanese had killed many Chinese. Among these victims, for example, were many stevedores done to death for not working hard enough. At that time, he was just a little boy, and it was difficult now for him to remember everything. I mentioned that it would be a good thing if one day the Chinese would be allowed to travel as we can. He said that he would like that very much and this would certainly be possible as soon as the socialist system in China had been fully established.

'Isn't it yet established then?' I asked.

'We'll still have to wait a little,' he said, evading the issue.

He looked at me from the side in a strange way, but said nothing more, and shook his head, whatever that may have meant.

If he were to come to Europe, I said, he could then take time off to learn a European language properly – English, for example. Here, that's not possible, I said, because there is no one who can really understand or speak European languages. On top of that, there were no proper language teachers. He could then one day teach European medical people in their own language, and as a result there would not be the many misunderstandings between students and their professors that there are now. At the moment, it is a total conceptual chaos and no one really understands what is meant and what the ancient classical texts imply.

Yes, he said, he would like to come to Europe very much indeed.

'Do you read a lot from the old classics?' he asked me as we walked along.

'Well, I originally learned Chinese from the new characters, but I have been trying for years to impress the classical characters on my mind, to analyse them and write them, and I do this with the help of a number of books.'

He was curious. Would it be possible, he asked, for me to show him the things I had learned? I was glad to oblige and took him up to the apartment. We sat down at the desk and grabbed some paper and a brush. I opened the book, *Huang-Di Su-Wen*, that I had just bought, and looked for the first chapter, *Shang-Gu Tian-Zhen*, which means 'On the Heavenly Truths Expounded by Our Forefathers'.

'We are concerned here about Shi, 時, Time,' I said. 'You know about this, I'm sure. Huang-Di asks his court doctor, Qi-Bo, about the possibility of lengthening human life and about maintaining health well into ripe old age. He receives the famous explanation concerning the time order of life with regard to men and women and that concerning the traditional virtues which govern the health of human beings.' I put my forefinger on the respective characters. 'These virtues are the Dao, 道, Yin-Yang, 陰陽, simple nutrition shi yin, 食飲, avoiding a foolish mind and too much exhaustion, bu wang zuo lao, 不妄作勞.'

Kang was nervous. He looked at the locked wall cabinet in our room, which began to rattle, especially when people were in the room. Achille and I were convinced that the room was wired up from that point. That was why we often spoke German or even Alsatian Low German.

I wrote down the ancient character for 'Time', Shi, 時. I knew this by heart, since it plays such an important role in medical literature.

'It shows the moving sun, 日, the growth, 生, of plants and animals in nature which it enables, and the individual human pulse in the character 寸; it can be found on the wrist. The ancient Chinese concept of time has to do with the human pulse and with the inner order of the individual, and this is very similar to the significance given to it by the pre-Socratic philosophers in ancient times in Europe. In modern China's abbreviated writing, the figure for "time" is given by 时, so that the idea of growth parallel with the movement of the sun is no longer to be seen. In former times, the human individual could grasp the idea of time and understand it by attending to his or her own pulse wave.'

Kang nodded, but said nothing.

'In the history of occidental thinking, Aristotle divided time into a number of intervals, small, individual sections similar to those which appear on the celluloid of a film strip.'

I wanted to go on with a more precise account of this, but he suddenly got to his feet. 'Shi?' he said absentmindedly, and then, 'Yes, Shi, Time. The term is important for China's old medicine.'

Kang's disquiet had deepened. The mention of 'time' in this context and in the various characters for the new and the old clearly irritated him.

'Xian-tsai Mei-you Shin-jian,' he blurted out. 'I've got no more time now!'

This meant that he suddenly had no more time to spend with me, and literally it meant 'no time gap'. The characters for this are shi jian, 時間.

Kang insisted that he had now to go home quickly. 'We'll see each other in the clinic tomorrow,' he added before he left.

The next few days further hindered our conversation about time, and he suggested that we carry on our discussion outside along the banks of the Huang-Pu River. So it came to be that we made special arrangements to see one another one evening at the river. I had the first volume of my book, the *Huang-Di Su-Wen*, with me.

'What's written there,' he said to me quietly, and after making sure that there was no one near to overhear us, 'is very dangerous.' His voice was hoarse. 'It contradicts the teaching of the Communist Party. In Mao's socialism, you see, there is no undivided flow of time and, especially, no difference between a man and a woman.'

'We know as doctors, though, that there is clearly a difference.'

Kang struggled for air. 'The Great Chairman Mao once said, and it's there for all to see in his red book, that men and women are identical. Same clothing, same haircut, and same money for same work.'

'But we know for sure that in reality both are quite different.'

'That's not true in modern China, except only under certain rare conditions.'

I could not help but laugh. 'Do you really believe that?'

To this Kang said nothing. He listlessly looked at the river moving along in the waning evening light.

'Look after your *Su-Wen* book carefully,' he advised me without looking my way. 'It's a miracle that you could have bought it at all, and clear, too, that the bookseller had no idea of what was politically correct.'

'You were there when I bought it', I said ingenuously. At this he stood up and wildly gesticulated with his arms. 'No, I was not there. You mustn't say that. I was never in that bookshop with you!'

For a horrible moment I thought he would snatch the book from me. But he was not so foolish as to do that. He knew that I was about to do something for him which was forbidden. I had brought a small present along with me for his children that I had bought at the Friendship Shop, a shop which he, as a Chinese, was not allowed to use. We had arranged that I would hand over the goods in a small thicket of wood not far from the harbour where no one would be able to see us.

'Should we go off to the wood now?' he asked. We both stood up and marched off in the direction of the Nanjing Road. He had made a plan.

'We'll go in different directions from here,' he announced. 'You go off towards the north side of the harbour to the wood and I'll approach from the south. There's only one way, and that leads through the wooded area. There, where it's really dark, we'll meet. Neither of us will say a word. We won't even look at each other, and we'll behave as if we didn't know each other. You give me that packet and I'll leave by the northern exit of the wood and you by the southern. If anyone is nearby when we approach each other, then we simply go on. No greeting. No stopping. The present will have to wait.'

There was no one in the little wood when we arrived. I looked up into the trees as I gave him the packet and he looked down to the ground. Neither of us looked at each other; neither of us said a word. From Nanjing Road I made my way directly back to the hotel. We had outwitted the ubiquitous spies.

Propaganda Films and Other Monkey Business

One day we watched a children's film in English called *The Red Star*. In it we learned of the destiny of a young man caught up in the struggle between the Red Army and the Guo-Ming-Dang. This young fellow stabbed a senior police officer who had formerly been a feudal lord. The policeman had had the boy's mother burned alive.

The film was pure propaganda; there were only very good people and very bad people in it. Violence was the order of the day. Children were encouraged to combat adults in an open war and with the help of pistols, fire, knives and hand grenades. All this was openly displayed in great detail. For me, the whole thing was morally reprehensible. Apart from that, the affair was kitschy, overblown and full of emotion, and the dialogue was inane and so silly that it was hardly bearable. People of flesh and blood just do not communicate in the way they did – not even in revolutionary China. The landscape in which all this took place was cardboard junk, and to propose such offensive rubbish for us to 'enjoy' was nothing short of insulting.

One of our Chinese colleagues from the university who had accompanied us praised the wretched thing in the highest tones. However, I wasn't having any of this, and opposed him by saying that the film was a shoddy, pitiful piece of ugly nonsense. We had, I added, seen better things here and certainly better films than this muck.

Adrienne, Alice, Achille and I went to see the famous Charlie Chaplin film *The Great Dictator*. It ran in the original English with Chinese captions, showing Adolf Hitler as a small Jewish hairdresser and as an arrogant despot. It was brilliantly portrayed as it dragged the latter through the dust of contempt. Achille suggested that all of us see the film and then 'we can see how the Chinese react to its content. After all, there are a hundred parallels between it and Mao Tse-tung's megalomania.'

During it, all four of us laughed at the parts we thought funny, but soon noticed that the Chinese laughed at quite different parts of the film. In fact, people turned round in their seats, annoyed with our laughter, and hush-hushed us to be quiet when we laughed at scenes where they were not amused. For our part, we could not understand why.

'I was pretty annoyed during the film,' Alice remarked as we walked back to the hotel. 'The other folks in the cinema had quite a different idea of what is funny than we did. I think they thought we were a group from outer space or something. Anyway, they think and feel quite differently, that's for sure. How can we ever come to understand one another?'

I keep thinking about the purpose of the hate-filled so-called Cultural

Revolution, which is still rampant in the country. It is the repression of the country's intellectuals – those people, that is, who could lead the country to something better than it is at the moment. Certainly there is method in Mao's madness. For when an entire people are repressed by fear and terror and also threatened with the death penalty, something that regularly takes place here during this 'Cultural Revolution', it is unlikely that anyone will insist on stating their own opinion.

When one frequently sees university professors with placards round their necks on which one reads 'I'm an idiot' or 'I'm an ass' led along Shanghai's Nanjing Road by Red Guards, with passers-by applauding this spectacle, one can well understand why people are not inclined to utter their own opinions. This is also the reason why this country has remained backward for so long, why such an inflexibly stupid, concrete form of socialism has developed in the country, why there is no intellectual activity, no creative initiative at work, and why there is no artistic expression. Apart from this, the fact is that many people are really badly off, and that is why they feel miserable and oppressed – their job just allows them to survive and no more. Whether this state of affairs can be justified historically is another matter. On the other hand, when a nation's people are held in existential terror, it is easy to govern them. In this respect, we in our democratic systems are much better off, since much is self-regulating. If one government makes a mess of regulating state affairs, then it has to withdraw, and then along comes another which exerts itself to do better. At least for a time. For that reason, there is no deep-seated fear infesting the individual in western countries; there is no violent repression. These things are something quite alien to people in those countries.

Is there anything, then, which is positive in China? It is tiresome always to have to report the worst of a country. Let's take the most elementary need of a person, that of having to live somewhere. Our hotel room was perfectly adequate. After all, the place was built by the British. But the living conditions of the people in the city are catastrophic. Most people live many to one room. The windows are almost always open. There is no heating system. Every day, the so-called street committee composed of completely alien people has to see if everything is 'politically in order'.

Life in the hotel was more or less bearable, except for the fact that the service was very bad. Although from a Chinese perspective, we lived in luxury, service personnel never knocked on the door, instead storming into the rooms screaming at each other like jungle birds, invading our private rooms, throwing things on the beds, disturbing us at unreasonable hours and moments. Happily, our respective toilets were lockable from the inside. At least we could withdraw to this one refuge to read or even to write.

It was quite impossible to receive a guest in the room without being disturbed or to read or write something in peace. There was always someone banging against the door and before you knew where you were, he or she was in the room without requesting entry. The younger hotel personnel were sullen and unfriendly. There was one on our floor who constituted the exception, greeting us and sometimes even smiling. It was mainly the older ones who, presumably, had learned European manners under the British who were different. An older waiter in the restaurant was especially kind, and another older staff member on the reception desk was friendly and polite. All the rest here were of the younger generation, brought up by the so-called people, so that they only knew bad manners. Apparently, this was the ticket to success in China's socialism, where a big mouth, brashness and sharp elbows together determined the standard of living.

We could see this in the case of our interpreters, where the tone of communication among them was rough and ready. In observing them, I was again and again reminded of the years of Nazi terror where coarseness, rudeness and the mindless repetition of party clichés determined the level of human intercourse, and where only above-average performance in sport brought recognition among young people, all of whom were more or less forcibly recruited into the ranks of ongoing soldiers and Nazis.

The next consideration was our meals. Although, compared with what the average Chinese eats, we were quite well nourished, the dishes all tasted the same. There were no deviations. We received no fresh vegetables, no salads, little fruit, and as a result fewer vitamins and no trace elements.

For us, the famous Chinese cuisine just did not exist any more, except perhaps where it could be found in the expensive restaurants lining Nanking Road. All our meals were prepared in fat, and the Canton rice, which we received each day, swam in a greasy broth into which a few eggs had been stirred. The drinks were always the same: Tsingtao beer and Lao-Shan mineral water. In the evening we sometimes drank a glass of their sticky-sweet red wine, the only wine to be found here.

The service in the restaurant was both unfriendly and repulsive. One waiter actually shoved his elbow into my rice bowl. This particular elbow had an inflamed, reddish-violet rash on it. When I objected, I received contempt, the fellow looking away in disinterest. Only when I adopted the same pointed rudeness as his did he deign to bring a fresh bowl, although I suspect it was exactly the same one as before. Two young waiters stood by me and watched me eat. They were greatly amused by the fact that this 'Long-Nose' did not want to partake of the 'elbow' rice. A number of us did not eat rice at all, but preferred noodles.

Aladin, the tall African from Chad, a man of few words and whom I had never seen laugh, once complained loudly about these awful meals. He had just eaten noodles which were hardly warm. At home in Africa, he said, he was far better nourished. Then he told us a story.

'I was once in Paris,' he began.

At this Achille and Adnan sang out, 'O-ho, Aladin, o-ho! In Paris!'

'Yessir! I was in Paris, and one evening I was walking along the Seine all on my own, you know, and what did I find there under a bridge? A dead man, a corpse. At first I thought he was just asleep, but when I moved him slightly with my foot, I saw straightaway that he was dead. He lay on his belly. I can quickly tell the difference between a dead man and one who's alive, you know.'

Everyone laughed.

'Well, Doctor Aladin, are you quite sure about that?' Achille asked in fun.

'Yes, I can,' Aladin said firmly. 'I went a little further along the river when suddenly I heard footsteps behind me. I looked around and what did I see? Two clochards were busy with the corpse. They had turned it over and were pressing the cadaver. From that distance I could hear them talking to each other quietly. They were hungry.

' "Do ye think he's got anything in his stomach?" the one asked.

' "Let's see," said the other and drew out a long knife. He slit the man's stomach open and looked inside.

' "Noodles," he said, "his last meal was noodles."

' "We could eat them," said the other, "after all, we haven't eaten anything for the last three days."

' "You can have them if you want," said the man with the knife.

"No, please, you eat them; I'll leave it for you to get on with it."

'It went on like this for a minute or two until one of them put his hand into the dead man's stomach and downed the noodles. But only a minute or two later he was sick. All the noodles came up onto the street.

'The other immediately ate what had been brought up – to the very last morsel. The other, seeing this, said, "Why didn't you tell me you were so hungry, I would have gladly let you eat them first!"

'While he wiped his mouth, the other replied, "Well, it's like this: I could never abide cold noodles!" '

Alice and Adrienne had long since risen from the table and left the company in disgust.

Aladin laughed loudly, his mouth wide open, and one could see not only his stumpy, wide-apart teeth and his pink tongue sticking out towards us, but also his uvula, visible behind his gums. He laughed and laughed, and naturally we all laughed with him.

When he had finished, he said, catching his breath at intervals, 'This just occurred to me when we were again eating them bloody noodles today.'

Systematic Clampdown on Education

I noticed here how my differentiated European thinking, my intellectual considerations, which were the basis for my western powers of reflection, were beginning to lose more and more impetus. I reacted only to the black-and-white standard patterns arising from the unpleasant impressions around me. The only area in which I found myself still capable of thoughtful criticism according to the norms of western standards was in my specialised area, medicine. Here, I was happy to be at the receiving end of the criticism and good humour of my surgeon colleague, Achille Haubensack, who had become an irreplaceable friend nearby with whom I could share my thoughts and feelings, and by whom I could also be corrected when necessary. However, I feared that the longer I stayed here, the more I would forfeit my intellectuality without really noticing its inexorable attrition.

The experiences I had with patients and with Chinese doctors in the clinic and at the university only served to strengthen this feeling of deterioration. China was capable of stultifying not only its essentially gifted people, but also its guests and visitors. If I did not have the daily luxury of being able to talk to my colleagues, I would have long since fallen into depression, frustration and desperation. The same was true of those students I had so far met who were studying in the People's Republic of China.

Today I was again in a bookshop. I wanted to buy as many medical works as possible for my library at home, and send them home by ship to Europe. This operation was made all the more difficult by the intervention of one of our interpreters, Xiao Gu, a mistrustful, moody individual who insisted on going with me to see what I was buying. In front of this very bookshop, she even attempted to prevent me from entering the shop by ordering the chauffeur to drive on straight back to the hotel.

I realised what she was doing and protested. Dr Kang, who happened to be with us, asked the driver to stop at the bookshop and to wait for us. This aroused Gu's fury and she gave vent to her opinions in a shrill, vitriolic outburst against Kang using the scolding tones of the marketplace. We got out at the bookshop nevertheless.

'Five minutes at the most are allowed for buying articles!' she shouted at us as we moved on. I turned round to correct her by quietly adding: 'You mean twenty minutes, don't you?'

But this Chinese harridan slammed the car door to and threw herself back against the car seat, sulking. While we were still looking for suitable books, this woman stormed into the shop and screamed at us, 'You're still not ready?'

'Xiao Gu, you are much too nervous,' I said. 'You are flapping and screaming around here. You'll be ill before you know what's what, and that would be a pity. Think of the traditions of Chinese medicine, of Yin and Yang, of the Dao and of your inner balance, which is the very basis of health.'

She laid great value on being called 'Madame', but I deliberately used her name, Xiao Gu, which means 'little woman' or 'Miss', and this annoyed her all the more. But the Chinese doctors also called her by the title 'Madame'. So why didn't I? She asked me several times to use her title, but I put her in mind of the fact that if she wished to be so addressed, then she should do something about her manners and so to live up to the title. Then, like any other French, Swiss or Dutch woman, for example, she would have earned it. But the truth was that she was a dyed-in-the-wool communist and a party member, and perhaps proud of the fact. For this reason, 'Xiao Gu' was the right title for her. After I had said this, she behaved a little better.

In the bookshop I acquired all the books that I wanted. It was quite simple. I went over to the shelves and selected the titles that interested me. Then I asked the bookseller to place the books on the counter for me to look at and finally choose. In this way, I came across a fine example of the book *Huang-Di Nei-Jing Ling-Shu*, another well-preserved example of *Su-Wen*, a *Shang-Han-Lun* and a *Jin-Gui Yao-Lüe*. In addition, I took a number of modern Chinese works on medical subjects, a handbook of internal medicine, a book on acupuncture and, lastly, a book on children's diseases and their cure.

Xiao Gu stood at the door with the driver, her otherwise so pale face now red with fury, muttering to herself. I behaved as if this uproar was all so much hot air. I paid and the bookseller put the books into a brown paper packet and tied it with string. I turned towards the door and saw the party woman showing her teeth to me. I glared at this little shrew and hissed, 'Zhu Kou!' ['Shut your mouth!'].

She shut up at once. We climbed into the car and drove back to the hotel in silence.

During my time in China, I noticed that those who were polite and used to what we call European manners were never treated seriously. Here, people had to be insolent to get what they wanted. Every party member used this ploy. Only those who had no advantage to gain or no axe to grind, or who were dependent, ill or weak in this ideologically contaminated land were friendly and polite. It was necessary, therefore, to have a few insulting phrases at hand to use like poisonous arrows in a quiver against people in conversation because, in keeping with Marxist dialectical tenets, other people could prove to be opponents and therefore needed to be kept at bay. This was an unpleasant situation that could never blossom into a peaceful exchange of opinion. It seemed as if there was a certain pecking order in the communist system, that operated according to the motto 'Those who can lash out best will be best respected'. Cheap vulgarity and impudence won the day here. It never worked to say, 'Would you be so kind as to . . .' or 'Could you perhaps please . . .', for this produced no effect at all. It was much better to roar your complaints out, make a stink, and brew a quarrel right from the start, otherwise you'd get nowhere. The best tactic was to stick your elbows in the ribs of others, to let them know immediately of your physical superiority. That was the everyday way of doing things in the land of 'comrades'.

The only polite Chinese person I knew in my near acquaintance was the ageing Dr Ou-Yang Shen, a relict from pre-revolutionary times that Mao's teaching had sought to violently root out by every means. I had the impression that this fine old gentleman suffered under China's current rule of the rabble. But nothing would change him; he was still one with his earlier good upbringing. As Europeans, we should constantly be aware of the fact that this brutalisation of China's proletariat was, finally, the product of our own western culture. It was the heritage of Marx, Engels, Lenin and Stalin which began with Russia and finally invaded a cultured and well-educated China to end up morally and spiritually poisoning its inhabitants. This 'new political line' had all its opponents interned in remote camps to the tune of hundreds of millions, then 're-educated' them there and finally murdered them by the million without conscience.

It was for this reason that people like Ou-Yang put up with the coarse reprimands coming from others such as Xiao Gu, Dr Kang and the interpreters without batting an eyelid. His face paled and the corner of his mouth turned down sadly. He was the one who was most friendly to his patients, and he was kind to children. He did not ram the needles into the flesh so brutally like the other Chinese medical staff who, without exception, were members of the Communist Party, otherwise they would not be allowed to have contact with us or to teach us. Dr Kang's technique with the needle was good, but his attitude to patients was incredibly rough and churlish, something I had myself experienced on catching a cold recently. His treatment hurt terribly and the results were minimal.

At dinner, I told my colleagues of my success at the bookstore. One or two of them said they would like to come with me on a general shopping tour.

Coarse and Fine Needle Techniques

Today we had a youngster in the clinic who had become hard of hearing after having suffered from a feverish illness, in this case probably meningitis. He shouted out so loudly in pain under Dr Kang's needle treatment that we feared the whole clinic would be alarmed by it.

Finally, the child's parents insisted he be treated by Dr Ou-Yang, and this Kang accepted with bad grace.

'Could it be that the treatment is ineffective when it causes so much pain to the patient?' I asked later.

Kang nodded without a word. I had the impression that many European acupuncture operators had a better technique than modern Chinese medical men, because they were more careful. It was not enough to have studied acupuncture in Chinese clinics. One must also have studied in European hospitals and studied western medicine and know it inside out. It was necessary to be acquainted with the western mentality, especially the European, since it was quite different from the Chinese.

I wanted on one evening to make another trip to a bookshop in Nanjing Street where I had seen a Chinese/English dictionary displayed in the window. Xiao Gu, who controlled our every movement, was as usual at my heels. She had wormed her way into the shop and, unbeknown to me, had exchanged a few words with the bookseller, who then told me that I could not buy the book. It was strictly for Chinese from a specific branch of professional activity.

'How come?' I asked.

Is it not highly desirable when we foreign friends wish to read and interpret the texts we study? After all, have we come here to study, have we not, and have sacrificed our time and our money for a good Chinese purpose. Sphinx-like, Dr Kang appeared in the entrance of the shop at this moment.

'You're here on a grant from the Chinese people,' the little witch Gu said sternly. 'That's why you have to do what we tell you. You have to obey our laws.'

As she said this, her face became an ugly mask. I contradicted her at once. 'On the contrary, I'm here on a German grant, put up by the German government.'

'You have received an offer of money from the Chinese state and you have accepted this money. As a result, you are subject to our conditions.'

Her face had become snow white with anger. I had for a long time expected such a situation to arise.

'I did not accept the offered stipend, but, on the contrary, returned it as a gift to the Academy for Chinese Medicine to buy teaching material,' I said. 'I am here with the scholarship from my own country, the Federal Republic of Germany, and I pay out for what I need in China from my own pocket.'

Xiao Gu doggedly persisted that I was paid by the People's Republic of China and had for this reason to subject myself to its regulations.

Dr Kang came up and intervened. He felt that Mrs Gu was right. I may not be allowed to buy the book.

'But, for God's sake, why?' I asked. 'If you know why, then you can tell me why!'

'I know perfectly well,' said Kang, 'but I'm not allowed to tell you. The party will not allow me to tell you.'

'So it's a state secret?'

'Yes,' said Kang.

What a state! And what a stupid party! I thought. What did it think it was doing with us foreign doctors? Were we just being abused for propaganda purposes? We were neglecting our clinics and losing money at home, and here we were learning nothing.

In response I then said that I would notify the chief organiser of the course, Dr Cai, from the Ministry of Health in Beijing, and ask him whether he would allow me to buy this dictionary. This was clearly a very uncomfortable suggestion for Kang. He said, feigning lack of interest, that I could do so if I really wanted to, but his face had become a mask of stone. His gesture froze as though he were a mime artist, and his body became a block of wood. It was at such moments that we saw the true blue party member who had sworn an oath of allegiance to the party and who would never infringe its principles, whereas, at other times, he was a friendly colleague. It was sort of an obsessional neurosis, a modern communist Chinese disease. Despite everything, I could not rid myself of the conviction that the main task of our Chinese colleagues was to hinder us from acquiring any knowledge of the deeper processes associated with Chinese medicine and acupuncture, and, above all, to prevent us from learning anything about needle analgesia in association with surgical operations. This prevention was what the party wanted.

Clearly, the party had its own secret plans for the dissemination of Chinese healing methods in the West. But what were these?

I had still been unable to buy the dictionary. But the next day I swung my leg over the saddle and cycled into Nanjing Road, went into the bookstore, got the book from the shelf, put it on the counter without a word, paid and left.

Not long before I was with Kang in the cinema. During the showing there was a scene in the film depicting a woman who was about to become a member of the Communist Party, and who was obliged to swear allegiance on the party's red flag. She had to swear that everything the party required from her would have priority over her family and even over her life. At this Kang was quite moved and leaned over to me, whispering, 'Now she is a member of the Communist Party; it's the holiest moment in her whole life!' He seemed to be deeply moved and had tears in his eyes. I said nothing, because I knew Kang would have never understood my views. The whole affair was similar to that of a nun entering a medieval cloister, Achille commented when I told him of my experience.

There was no one in our group who would not be pleased when the course came to an end. No one would want to stay on for any reason. All of us were fed up to the back teeth. Even the political leftists in our company, above all the younger doctors such as Reto Armbruster, the Laotians and the men from Cameroon, were of this opinion.

Today a letter arrived from the Dutch embassy in Beijing to the effect that the First Secretary had been actively looking after our interests with regard to acupuncture anaesthesia at the Ministry of Health in Beijing, where it had been made clear that we as western doctors would not be allowed to practise this kind of anaesthesia for reasons related to the responsibility accorded to doctors in China. According to this letter, the fact was that we were guests in the People's Republic and as such were obliged to conform with that which was offered for us to study. We were not in a position to insist on bilateral agreements in this connection and were obliged to accept that which was freely taught to us. I was reminded of talks with the secretary of state at the Ministry of Health in Bonn, who had reported that the German Federal Republic did indeed have such bilateral agreements with the People's Republic of China for training German doctors in China and Chinese doctors in West Germany.

At least this agreement was official in my own case, and so what had been stated by the Chinese authorities here was simply not true. However, I do not know whether this was applicable to all my fellow colleagues.

Something Afoot in Needle Analgesia

The reality, however, seemed to be slightly different. Early one morning, we eighteen doctors were invited to watch the process of needle analgesia at work, not, it was emphasised, to practise it. To this end, we found ourselves standing around an operating table which, of course, did not allow optimal observation for us to learn anything.

In Europe, we would know what to do about such a situation. We would know to whom to apply. We would ring the appropriate ministry and ask how the thing should be solved. If we would like this or that, something would happen in our countries. We were all of us experienced professionals and chosen by our respective governments as suitable candidates for further training in China. We could not allow ourselves to sit around and do nothing. But here, no one knew to whom to apply. The business was like finding yourself in an opaque, impenetrable jungle thicket, among a stifling, defeating undergrowth of nescience. No one knew who the man of the moment was who could make the appropriate decision in this case. We had to rely on a subsidiary group of people for the answers, and this was particularly upsetting for European citizens, academicians and democrats alike.

Instead of answers we were given a diversion for the masses: after the evening meal, we had to go to a puppet theatre performance in which – how could it ever be otherwise? – the 'Gang of Four' were presented as the enemy of the state and of mankind in general. As in the classic Chinese opera, little bells jingled and big gongs droned. Shrill Chinese voices shrieked party-political slogans such as, 'Si-Ren-Deng [Gang of Four]!' These dreadful criminals, one of whom (interestingly enough) was Mao's wife, how wicked they were! Again and again. But the whole performance was utterly boring and patently stupid, a huge stir about nothing. At the end, these traitors were condemned by little children, and the masses carried the maltreated dolls away in triumph from the stage. The brainwashed mob was enthralled. Was this a kind of vent for their subconscious aggression that simmered below the surface of a repressed people? Behind the puppet show, the oversized heads of Mao and Hua Guo-Feng could be seen all the time.

Performances of this kind did little to make our stay more pleasant. The marionette management was gauche and insensitive in comparison with the grace and charm of the Salzburg puppet theatre to be seen from time to time in the Mozart operatic performances held in that city. And as far as new Chinese music was concerned, one could only say that its 'western-style revolutionary' character was noisily violent, full of screeching vocalists and intrusive rattling and drumming. In this most primitive way, Shanghai children were inculcated into believing that all foreigners and old people were mere relics of an earlier time that was rich in tradition, and that they were in fact enemies of the state and, for that reason, traitors and therefore must be eradicated. This notion turned former Chinese tradition upside down. Whereas at one time, age was honoured and a long life regarded as a virtue in China, today old people and foreigners were subjected to the most humiliating, most degrading and disgraceful treatment by Chinese children in such a show.

Surprisingly, my bicycle, which had gone astray, turned up at the hotel again after I had declared that it had been stolen, a phenomenon that is practically non-existent in today's China. Two of our interpreters brought it along and gave the following explanation for its temporary loss: Red Army soldiers had discovered the machine standing outside a bookstore in Nanjing Road where I was making my purchases. It was not locked, since this was not necessary in the 'Land of the Good Chinese'. Hair-raising penalties were dispensed for theft, including, not infrequently, the death penalty. As a consequence, my bicycle was transferred to a nearby yard for safety. There was a 'no parking' order that was applicable to cycles in Nanjing Road. The soldiers felt that I would eventually find my bike in the yard after a thorough search. The truth was that I would have done no such thing. Instead, I alerted the city police – which is what I did – and certainly a most thorough search of the neighbourhood from top to bottom ensued, they said. They had found the bike and found out somehow that the bike, a fine black affair and one of the best bikes I have ever owned, belonged to me. It still stood where they had placed it in the yard behind the bookshop. Nothing gets lost in China, at least not in today's Shanghai.

Yesterday morning I was again in Nanjing Road, this time to procure enough paper to wrap my books in, and again I found myself surrounded by a stupid crowd of curious onlookers. I wanted to get through them to the shop and cried something like 'Boo-boo-boo' or 'Wei-wei-wei' at them, but they stood there like a wall looking at me as though I had just fallen from the moon. Finally, I reached the stationery shop (the same emporium I had visited a few weeks before to acquire a brush), bought what I wanted, and in the afternoon packed my books and took them to the post office. The packet had to be examined by officers of the post authority, and each book was punctiliously scrutinised. Three books were not permitted, since, apparently, they were only for distribution in inland China.

Two were works concerning old techniques in pulse diagnosis and one was on the theme of Qi-Gong, a therapy similar to that of Tai-Chi-Quan involving exercises and breathing techniques to combat numerous diseases, including cancer. I took these three books back with me to the hotel, and the rest I sent by registered post to Germany. While I was involved in this protracted investigation of purchases, which, incidentally, took all of two hours, there was a violent altercation between two Chinese men at a neighbouring counter. I had never seen anything like it before in China. They screamed at one another, kicked out at one another and pulled at each other's hair. Those standing around tried to separate these two furious fighting cocks, but had their work cut out to achieve anything at all. In general, Chinese folks are patient and peaceful, so it is pretty certain that it was a deeper cause than usual that had brought them to the boil, and probably one concerned with neurotic or psychopathic pressure.

Back at the clinic one morning I had difficulty once again with our interpreter 'Madame' Gu – always referred to by me as Xiao Gu, 'Little Gu'. She was an intelligent person, but someone who was evidently bored with the work given to her involving the translation of medical texts and the control of foreign doctors. She not only irritated the European doctors, but also managed to vex our Chinese colleagues with insinuations and unfriendly gestures. The Chinese put up with it all because she had an important function at the Ministry of Health in Beijing, was therefore often sent abroad on confidential missions, and her father was supposed to be a prominent communist and party member. She, however, had quite unacceptable habits. She constantly interrupted exchanges between Dr Kang and myself, and I took the opportunity to ask her whether she was there to interpret or to block the flow of scientific information between us physicians. She took no notice of this whatsoever.

'If you were to take more trouble about correct translation,' I told her, 'the quality of instruction in general would be a lot better. On the whole, you interpret wrongly. Do you want to keep us in the dark on purpose? We know very well in Europe what Chinese medicine is, so we don't need your assistance.'

At this she burst into a tirade of hate and venom.

Finally, I said to her, 'Now interpret quickly and above all correctly what my Chinese colleagues say to you!' She was clearly nervous at this, because she wasn't capable of doing so. She sat for a whole hour and sulked, during which we were able to happily chat with our teachers.

As a matter of interest, the Chinese system of health is not the rosiest, as is often maintained in the West. If someone falls ill, the first thing that is done is to deduct thirty per cent from his salary, and then, on top of that, he will have to pay for treatment. In the morning, he will have to draw an entrance ticket from the reception at the clinic dealing with his particular treatment. Treatment is therefore not so cheap when one considers what a worker earns each month. Intellectuals do not earn much more than workers. Members of the party, however, receive much more money. Reckoned in German marks and in terms of European purchasing power, a consultation at a clinic costs around 20 euros.

It may be true that socialism is much talked about here in red China, but in Western Europe at least 'socialism' has long been realised, and our health system is better by a long chalk. What, for example, would happen if we too were to deduct thirty per cent from a worker's wage when he falls ill? The unions would get on their hind legs and stage an impressive demonstration. From a European point of view, one could say: 'In China, everyone talks about socialism, but we in Europe have it!' Achille and I were never tired of proclaiming this. 'Let's not forget that when we get back home,' he warned me.

The Meaning of Food

The most important topic in China is without doubt that of food. What at first may seem to be a primitive preoccupation is not in fact so. Food, like good medicine, is life promoting. So it is that two Chinese doctors can talk for hours about 'Chi-Fan' – that is, about eating rice.

This usually takes the following form: 'What did you eat yesterday?' In answer, a comprehensive description of all the food eaten the day before is reviewed for the questioner. 'What do you think we'll have to eat today?' A list of all the most desirable dishes usually provides an answer.

'Are we too early for the meal, do you think?'

'We could come too late.'

'We mustn't do that! Better finish work a bit earlier!'

Then the two doctors go over to the wardrobe to check the cups and plates they are carrying with them. Safety first. In doing so, the crockery must be tapped with chopsticks, because this produces an 'atmosphere of cheerfulness'. Next to Communist Party membership, eating occupies a position of highest priority in the lives of mainland Chinese.

Lunch is served every day at 12 noon sharp. Three years ago, I had booked a flight from the Li River to Shanghai. During the trip from Gui-Lin to Shang-Sha, I heard that the pilot had asked over the intercom whether before finally landing at our destination it might not be possible to make a stopover somewhere for lunch. All the passengers thought this was a great idea. The pilot then enquired if it was possible to land at a little airport en route where there was plenty of food, and this was exactly what he did, touching down at a small airport and we later filed into a restaurant full of hungry Chinese. After this, it was necessary to take a short nap ('Xiu-xi'), so the two pilots settled themselves among the cushions in the waiting hall and slept on them with wide-open mouths for the next fifteen minutes. After they woke up, the journey continued. As a consequence of this holy 'Chi-Fan', I missed my connecting flight to Shanghai and had to spend a boring night in some remote place in the countryside.

We, too, were beginning to acquire the 'Chi-Fan' mentality for the simple reason that there was nothing else going on here. We were somehow miraculously changed to the negative in-out mentality. As a result, Achille and I looked forward to our evening beer like children do to Christmas. Both of us found this metamorphosis a matter for serious reflection and introspection. Could it be that we'd shortly have nothing more in our heads than 'Chi-Fan' and Tsing-tao beer? I mentioned to Achille that this food obsession could be a symptom of a regrading of our minds to an infantile level. It is well known that for children and animals, meals and food are the most important things. Sigmund Freud, the psychanalyst, has dubbed that period in human life the 'oral phase'. Were we in fact already retrograded to such a primitive mental state?

Here in China, there is otherwise nothing to do; indulging in hobbies or owning anything other than a few personal belongings is not permitted. It is of course possible to swim against the current, but before long, other Chinese would notice what was going on, report these activities to the revolutionary committee, who, in their turn, would notify the street committee, and a little after that, neighbours would come along to publicly denounce you. I had actually been witness to one of these communal denunciations in the Hua-Dong Hospital when, accidentally, I stepped into a wrong room. The room itself was totally dark, but beyond it, in another room I could hear an appalling hubbub of female voices raised in anger. I managed to peek through a gap of the door. In the middle of this gesticulating, screaming, hellish commotion stood a young woman in a blue dress and white blouse on a stage, her eyes bloodshot with crying, her head sunk on her chest, surrounded by an aggressive mob of women waving their fists and pointing their fingers at her while others even spat at her. Apparently, the poor creature had done something to contravene party regulations and so deserved public humiliation. As the room I stood in was in complete darkness, no one could have seen me, so I stayed for about twenty minutes and then slipped out without notice. Foreigners are not permitted to be party to such degrading scenes.

VII

Is a New Revolution Necessary?

One of the worst things about this country is that in the name of socialism and communism, human dignity is trampled underfoot. As I mentioned a moment ago, the individual has no claim to anything he can call his own. He must sacrifice all he has – and sometimes, if thought necessary, his very life – for the party. He has become the slave of the state, with all that this implies. And if it were not for the fact that we were guests of the Chinese state, we would with certainty have been treated the same way – like animals or worse.

Since there is nothing here above the mundane, nothing higher than the ordinary such as, for example, an honourable approach to life or noble cultural objectives in the European sense, most people revert to what is left – eating. There is no alternative that would somehow make life worth living, and intellectual impoverishment is here beyond compare. As a result of this vacuum, nothing develops from this mental bankruptcy. There is only an arid landscape of stupidity and brutality, a common denominator of animal brutishness that is quite simply opposed to the development of human nature.

The question is: just how long will China tolerate this? At some time or other, people will rise up and say 'No' to the burdens laid upon them. At some time there has to be a revolt against the present regime. One can only hope that such opposition will come into being peacefully and constitute a harmonious development in line with the current economic potential of this country and the rest of the world. The results of a violent uprising would be catastrophic.

The average Chinese is quite ready to talk about his ancient culture, but he himself is kept in ignorance about it, and is not personally capable of any cultural achievement. He is not encouraged to go to school for longer than prescribed, and this can easily be seen in the miserable standards of instruction, including medical instruction, at universities. The Shanghai College of Chinese Medicine, which today is a university, is no exception. Anyone who has studied at a European university and acquired his or her degree there and later comes to China can quickly substantiate this. What for the moment artificially protects communist China like its Great Wall from international exposure is, for the most part, its impenetrable language. With regard to the many opacities of the language and the ambiguity of its written characters, one has to admit that everything can actually mean something completely different from what is generally accepted!

Here, one can get along nicely in this thoroughly false, mendacious society with its pretty party slogans, plenty of ugly elbows and impudence. I experienced this every day when, as a state guest, I found it necessary to correct interpreters, but it was only in this way that one could engender respect and achieve what it was necessary to achieve – namely, to be better informed about Chinese medicine. In supplying us with the means to acquire this knowledge, the interpreters were crude in their solutions and primitive in their behaviour. They very well knew the rules of their party-political, over-organised society where they could bamboozle others with their ostensible superiority, but in terms of blunt fact, they had almost nothing to offer us.

So it is that the reality in this country is diametrically opposed to that which its socialist programme purports to want to achieve. This red socialist republican reality has proved to be the exact opposite of its theoretical basis. Its inner contradiction would have secretly pleased the 'Great Chairman', Mao Tse-tung, because, had he lived long enough, he would have seen himself confirmed as having unified the opposites!

Acupuncture Analgesia on Human Guinea Pigs?

We were in the gynaecological department today and were allowed to witness a number of acupuncture analgesia procedures. We could see in general that these operations were conducted with great care, so that the patient did not experience pain. For this reason they lasted roughly twice as long as those carried out in western orthodox clinics.

The surgical problems involved are in general as follows:

1. The acupuncture analgesia is still underdeveloped.
2. The relaxation of the muscles is inadequate.
3. Where the surgeon sees the need to pull at the intestines, the patient experiences much dull, heavy pain.

In principle, it can be asserted that the simplest operations are on the throat, and that the face and the head are most effective to anaesthetise, because here the path to the brain is shorter, and it is here, too, that in the brain (in the thalamus and hypothalamus), the body's own pain-relieving substances, such as endorphins and enkephalins, are released.

The first patient received a ligature of the fallopian tubes to prevent further pregnancies; she already had a daughter, and that was deemed enough for a modern Chinese mother.

I said to Alice, the Dutch paediatrician, who was standing next to me, that I could well imagine that in future women like this one would one day make it possible to do without children altogether, and this was completely opposed to the Chinese policy during pre-communist times.

'Has there ever been something like this in Germany?' she asked me.

'No. In Germany's Nazi period, mothers of more than three children were awarded a cross of distinction, the "Mother's Cross", because they had provided the "Führer" with more welcome cannon fodder or had proved themselves worthy of providing more soldiers and party members. My grandmother, for example, had brought four children into the world and consequently was awarded an appropriate medal by the local Nazi officials for 'enriching the Reich'. The award went up in flames together with her house and property in 1944 during an allied night raid. Despite the war and the Nazi reign of terror, the four children survived. Two of them were lucky enough to move to the United States in time and to lead happy and healthy lives there, and that was the main thing.'

'Many female doctors in Europe have not enough time to procreate and to raise children,' Alice said.

Adrienne, as an expert in the techniques of anaesthesia, very carefully followed the procedures used throughout the operation. 'Well, it's just different here,' she said, and then went on to add, 'this is a comparatively simple operation and it is sufficient to stimulate both San-Yin-Jiao (spleen 6) points, which lie above the ankle on the inner side of the leg. These sites are combined with three points at the ear – namely, the points Shen Men (ear 55), the lungs (ear 101) and the uterus (ear 58). All these ear structures are punctured and then electrically stimulated.'

The placement of the needles and the electric stimulation of these had begun fifteen minutes before the operation. The patient felt very little of what was going on, and in twenty minutes the operation had been successfully brought to a conclusion.

We were also present at a normal birth, which took place under the influence of needle analgesia. Here, too, the points San-Yin-Jiao (spleen 6) and He-gu (large intestine 4) on both hands were used, and with these, labour can be induced, although during pregnancy of the earlier months, this is something which must be strictly avoided, so as to avert the possibility of a miscarriage. Incidentally, from time to time, these points are in fact used in China to facilitate abortion. However, their employment only brings about an incomplete abortion and one that has to be eventually fully realised by surgical intervention in the form of a curettage procedure.

There followed a so-called D&C (dilation and cauterisation of the cervix) on a 42-year-old patient, and here the same points were used as in the operations described above. The patient felt no pain during the 15-minute procedure.

After this, we watched a hysterectomy, the removal of the womb. Adrienne made her own notes on this: 'Needles were placed forty minutes before the operation. They were set at the following sites: Yao-Shu, a point at the upper end of the anal fold; Ming-Men (governing vesse 4) at the fourth lumbar vertebrae; Dai-Mai (gall bladder 26) at the anterior end of the free eleventh rib; Zu-San-Li (stomach 36) at the upper, anterior shin bone muscle; San-Yin-Jiao (spleen 6), a hand's breadth above the ankle, and finally, Ci-Liao (bladder 32), in the 2nd foramen of the sacral bone.'

During these preparations the patient lay for ten minutes on her side, then she was carefully placed on her back. The electrical stimulation was continued during the whole course of the operation.

The surgeon, a strong, muscular woman, first of all tested the insensitivity of the lower abdomen, then opened up the skin in an arc-like incision, the so-called panhandle incision, about 10 centimetres long. The subcutis and abdominal muscle were exposed and severed. Now the operational area was open to view. The parametrium, ligaments and fallopian tubes were separated and split on both sides of the uterus.

The patient had already begun to moan as the peritoneum was cut open. When the ends of the parametrium were sewn, the woman let out a shrill cry of pain. The veins of the uterus were ligamented and the woman cried out even more. She pleaded for a normal, full anaesthetic, but the Chinese surgeon and her assistants denied her this. A nurse kept waving Mao's red bible in front of the patient's face for quite a while, but the poor woman kept her eyelids tightly closed in unbearable pain. The procedure was a slow one in order to spare the patient unnecessary pain, but, despite this, the whole business was a long, torturous struggle for her.

The uterus was pulled up from the body cavity and the blood vessels cut, an operation which caused the poor woman extra agony. Her pain seemed not to influence anybody in the slightest.

Adrienne was appalled. 'Is this what they mean by "serving the people"?' she asked. 'The whole affair is just barbarous!'

The anterior vaginal wall was then separated and the vagina cut. The woman screamed even louder and began to twitch. This only complicated the situation. The round ligaments on the stump of the cervix were sewn together. This took more than half an hour. The question troubling us all was how long the hapless woman could hold out? The pain was apparently becoming too much for her, and she could well die of shock while on the operating table. Finally, she was fitted with a drainage tube at the cervix. The sewing up of the wound took an age. The peritoneum was closed and the abdominal muscles were sewn closely together. Lastly the skin of the patient was closed. She was clearly at the end of her resources and certainly this operation had been infinitely more strenuous than any formal anaesthetic would have rendered it. It would leave the woman traumatised for the rest of her life.

'No!' Alice cried in indignation. 'That's not any kind of progress in medicine!' Having watched the procedure to the end, this Dutch pediatrician, horrified by what she had just witnessed, went out to be sick.

Adrienne had carefully observed everything with dismay, and said later, 'One shouldn't forget that this process is not so much proper anaesthetics, but more what we would call hypalgesia or a reduction of sensitivity to pain. The operation as a consequence takes far longer to complete than it would using normal, western techniques – often up to four times as long. An experienced surgeon in the West needs about an hour for a hysterectomy, but here this took four hours, and for all this time the patient was subjected to dreadful pain. We were eyewitnesses to the drama from beginning to end. It contradicts the simplest basic rules of medical endeavour!'

Achille said contemplatively, 'Another contradiction within Mao's kingdom? A beastly example. To the devil with all this communist bullshit!'

Once we had returned to the hotel, all of us discovered that we had no appetite. Instead, we sat in the room next to the restaurant and discussed what we had seen. The surgeon, Walo Sifferlin, took up the theme.

'The poor woman had groaned and screamed, and had asked the doctors to ease her pain, but despite that, she had to go through four hours of torture. With a modern injection she would have felt nothing at all. The question is whether this four-hour exposure to intense pain was not at the same time a disturbance of the general circulation, the stability and balance of all the patient's other organs and much more of a strain to her than a normal, full anaesthetic. As western doctors, we have to view this method of analgesia with a very critical eye before it is presented to the world as something of a breakthrough. Red China at the moment is misguiding the world with a gigantic fraud. In the West, our medical and ethical principles would never allow us to put a patient to such a test.'

Mahmud Atassi added that it was now probably unlikely that we would be shown any more operations using needle analgesia.

Adnan Kirinin said thoughtfully, 'The first operations were simple and went off better for that reason. The ligaturing of the fallopian tubes to sterilise the woman made use of an effective form of anaesthesia by attaching needles to the ear and to the leg and then stimulating them electrically. That indeed was interesting. The ear needle was directly connected to an electrical device and the patient received no pre-medication, or at least no one mentioned it if they were. Apparently, such an operation is possible under these conditions.'

Achille chipped in, 'One can't undertake big operations using this kind of method, let alone not anaesthetise patients sufficiently. They're just not manageable like that. It means the surgeon has to work very slowly, and this fact alone is something of a torture for the patient. We at home like to work quickly in order to keep the whole affair to a minimum time, but on this occasion everything went at a snail's pace so as not to damage the peritoneum and the intestines, but as the uterus was removed, the woman suffered great pain on the table; she threw her head from one side to another and waved her arms about and screamed. One just can't put anyone through that torture!'

I added sarcastically, 'Oh yes we can, dear colleagues – in this paradise of farmers, soldiers and workers, it's not only possible, it's the duty of a communist hero.'

'Yes, like the medical tests on human beings in Nazi concentration camps,' Achille commented.

'The closed ranks of the masses evidently demand such victims,' said Jean-Claude Giroudou. 'All the more praise for our Christian Occident!'

Only Babu and Aladin had in the meantime acquired an appetite and returned to the dining room to find something to eat. The rest of us went out into the fresh air.

Back in our apartment, Achille said maliciously, 'I remembered during the beastly operation that I once read a sarcastic pamphlet written by the English writer Swift, the author of *Gulliver's Travels*, about reducing the vast number of poor Irish children in the seventeenth century. Swift was a clergyman and certainly in a very bitter mood when he proposed to feed these children to rich gentry people in England in order to let the Brits enjoy an especially delicious and rare meal prepared of these children provided they were young and well nourished.'

'You better stop telling me such ghastly things,' I said.

We had no appetite for drinking beer that evening either, but just ordered tea and mineral water.

Not Much Success with Needles. Why?

Just a word or two about the results of needle therapy. Quite a number in our group were very disappointed because they were not able see as many cures as they had hoped for. For my own part, and as far as our hospital was concerned, I can say that the success quota was quite good and corresponded more or less with the results reached at home. However, in saying this, it is necessary to add that any doctor who makes this claim must himself have acquired a certain self-assurance and experience before he can say as much.

Up to now, I had not learned a great deal. Spectacular results could not at all be accredited to acupuncture, and this applied even more so to 'wonderful' results. Anyone practising acupuncture is not a miracle worker, and that is really the first thing that has to be emphasised in the West. Often enough, there is also a need for a great many individual treatments, and it is also frequently necessary to augment these with Chinese herbs and with an honest personal consultation. What up to now has passed for 'acupuncture' in the West is merely an enormous swindle for patients and the public alike, and this must be corrected. The loud-mouthed advocates of acupuncture must be silenced for the simple fact that their enthusiasm is out of place and unjustified. Patients have only too freely been promised wonders – miracles that are medically quite impracticable.

Apropos of this, I have to mention a woman with tinnitus by way of example who has undergone treatment on five occasions. She is also suffering from sleeplessness and is very nervous. Now, she sleeps better and her nervousness has been ameliorated, but the noise in her ears remains. Many patients with stomach problems have been cured, and several children with digestive problems have been healed completely.

I talked recently with Albert Lagarde about the patient with hearing trouble. He looked at me slightly askance. 'Shall I tell you something, Ralf?' he began. 'We have no chance with her. She is suffering from something quite different from "kidney emptiness", which is her official Chinese diagnosis. Old Ou-Yang whispered it to me during treatment the other day. Her son was hauled out of bed one night by Red Army soldiers and taken away. Since that time she's heard nothing of him and has fallen ill. Since then her ears have been ringing.'

'What did her son do to earn that?'

'Probably transgressed some party rule or other – it's so easy!'

'How right you are! Perhaps he has been wearing a western tie or peeping into old books or perfumed himself. Or perhaps he had even possessed photos of pretty Chinese girls, and some "comrade" has denounced him.

Anyway, one thing's true: this woman has been suffering from tinnitus since the shock of her son's arrest.'

'Arbitrary arrests in the early hours were part of the Nazi horror in Germany,' I said.

'We French folks only knew about that during the occupation. What was it like in Germany?'

'I recall being on my way to school one morning with a lad from the neighbourhood, when we lived in Emden's Achterdiek. We used to walk along Uferstrasse on our way there. His name was Frithjof, and he was a year older than I was and owned a wristwatch. I could always ask him the right time. Anyway, one morning he didn't want to go with me. He took a long route via another street and from there eventually turned into Uferstrasse, where we came across each other again.

' "What's up?" I asked him. He stared at the ground.

' "My father said I shouldn't tell anybody, but I'll tell you. My mother was taken away tonight."

' "Who took her away?"

' "I can't tell you that either," said Frithjof.

'His father was a harbour pilot and highly respected, an important man in the town's community and esteemed among ships' personnel. For this reason, he was not expected to do military service. My father knew him well. Frithjof was their only child.

' "Tell me, please," I pleaded. He looked desperate.

' "My mother is Jewish," he said, "and that's why she was taken away," he muttered. "And that's why I mustn't go along with you on the pavement to school. They told me. I'm half Jewish."

' "Such rot," I replied. "We know each other so well, Frithjof, and I want to go to school with you, and what's more I'm going to. You've got the watch, what time is it? Are we going to get there on time?"

' "It's still only ten to eight," Frithjof replied, somewhat relieved.

'From then on, we went to school together as before. A few weeks later, he told me that his father had fallen ill. "He's not eaten anything for days and is terribly thin."

'I remembered Pilot Poppinga as a well-built Frieslander. "What's the matter with him?" I enquired.

' "It's just that my mother's no longer there," Frithjof said. "He goes out in our boat in the evening and rows out to the Dollart. He knows his way about of course. A few days ago he went as far as Lütje Horn. I was glad to see him back at night. He tells me he's got a noise in the ears all the time since my mother left."

'Herr Poppinga then became seriously ill. No one, it seemed, could help him. He finally lost his job, because the party wanted it that way. Just before the end of the war he died in an asylum near Oldenburg. I don't know what happened to Frithjof.'

'That's a dreadful reminiscence, Ralf,' said Albert Lagarde.

Achille remained sceptical as far as Chinese medicine was concerned. He did not believe in the existence of the 'meridians', and compared belief in them to the silly belief some people entertain with regard to religion, which he didn't believe in either. 'That's all a lot of childish nonsense, and we're out of this infantile stage,' he would say. Then I repeated what I had said on our first evening together in Beijing.

'The Chinese character for "meridian" is something quite different from that which we are told; I've already made that clear to you. There are no "meridians" in Chinese medicine. The idea stems from a glaring error in westerm translation.'

He did not believe me. He didn't believe anything that was said to him any more. 'We're living among a pack of idiots,' he concluded, shaking his head.

'Who knows, perhaps you'll become a passionate supporter of acupuncture when you get home,' I said.

'Never on your life!' he said. 'Before that the Moselle River will flow backwards into the Vosges Mountains, my lad.'

I tried irony. 'My dear Doctor Haubensack. You have now been the guest of the Chinese government for two and a half months in the beautiful city of Shanghai. You ought to be able to say that acupuncture has quite revolutionised our modern medicine.'

Achille swallowed the desire to laugh out loud. He would have to first try acupuncture out on all his patients at home before he could sing its praises.

There is, however, one thing to add, and that is that the old theory as it appears, for example, in the 800-page Chinese standard work *Zhen-Jiu Xüe* is not at all adequate for western doctors as a means of understanding acupuncture. I mentioned this fact to Dr Kang, who suggested that we retire somewhere to quietly discuss the whole thing in confidence. Later, he came up to the hotel room again for this purpose.

I told him that if he wanted to 'sell' this type of medicine to Western doctors, he would have to make it much more attractive to them and also supply an underlying theory that was reasonable. 'Otherwise, it's no go,' I added.

A little abashed by this, he nevertheless agreed with me. I had seen the same problems three years ago, and had returned to Europe from China with many critical thoughts and comments – more, in fact, than I had imagined. And that was the way it was this time, too. I would go back home much more sobered than I had come.

Above all, I would have to add that the Chinese were linguistically too clumsy to really make themselves clear. Added to this was the fact that there were very few people who were properly educated from the scientific point of view. There were so-called professors who were to teach us what they knew. These were little more than adolescents with very meagre medical training and background, and who had no idea of the world of modern medicine in the West. Scientifically, they could be said to have had no training at all, and this fact alone had brought Chinese acupuncture into a difficult situation. To all intents and purposes, there was no one here who was qualified to elucidate this very interesting area in scientific terms and concepts. Generally, all interest seemed to centre on eating and political humbug.

I Do a Bit of 'Espionage'

After colleagues had gone off to play a bit of ping-pong, I decided to go to the Friendship Store on my own to fetch the silk shirts that the tailor had sewn for me. However, they were not my taste and not properly sewn either, and I asked him to correct this and measure me properly. I noticed that someone was watching me – a woman who looked like Xiao Gu. The next morning the interpreter Xiao Gu came up to me in a fluster and asked me unpleasantly where I had been in the evening.

'What are you up to so late at night in the dark streets of Shanghai alone?' she asked.

'Have you seen me there?' I enquired, and she answered, 'Yes.'

At first I refused to speak to her more, but as she insisted, I laid my hand just in front of her mouth and whispered, 'Je fais l'espionnage!'

She jumped back at this as though struck by lightning. Apparently, she believed my little joke. I had made the remark because I was fed up with this constant surveillance, this low-minded interference in other people's lives. Like the others of her ilk who had been party politically brainwashed by constant, inexorable indoctrination, she had become a rather pathetic figure, quite unable to understand others, and especially those from the West.

She pulled an evil face and warned, 'If you're indulging in espionage, you'll find yourself having to deal with us, the party. Our authorities are not going to put up with that, you can be sure!'

With that, she ran from interpreter to interpreter, from the Chinese doctors to the professor, and told them all of the wickedness of my ways. My silly joke, an expression of exasperation with this unbearable way of life, had become a punishable truth.

'These western doctors, especially this Mr Rompard and the French fellow' (Achille had immediately cottoned on to the catchword 'espionage'), 'belong to the opposition, and are therefore to be regarded as our people's enemy. The best thing to do is to observe them by day and night.'

Thus it was that the word 'espionage' hung like an omen in the air. Afternoons in the clinic were deadly boring. Everyone, including the Chinese doctors, yawned with fatigue at temperatures of almost 40°C. Even the gentlemanly old doctor Ou-Yang yawned luxuriously as the afternoon wore on. We did not know what to do with ourselves. This China had just become too monotonous. Then Xiao Gu, still alarmed by what I had uttered, took me to task again: 'Right, out with it! What were you doing all alone in Shanghai last night?' Her rudeness stank.

'Well, if you want to know, I was out with a very beautiful young woman.'

Xiao Gu hissed in disbelief. 'C'est impossible! There's no such thing as that here.'

'Why is it impossible?' I asked. 'People like me are up to that kind of thing all over the world. Women are women and men are men. In China, too. Is that not so? Do you want me to go into the differences in medical detail? I mean, purely in the interests of scientific investigation? You're a medical translator and all the appropriate vocabulary should be in your little dictionary or in your head.'

Xiao Gu showed no interest in my offer, but instead indignantly informed those Chinese standing around that I had gone out with a pretty Chinese woman on the evening before, and that was an insult to the propriety of Chinese womankind, whereupon she went into every neighbouring room of the study groups and told them that I had gone out with a Chinese the night before. That, she declared, was the very height of shamelessness, immorality, pornography, and was in every way unheard of! In all this, I heard a certain undertone which contained the following question: 'How can this Western subhuman dare to say anything that would compromise Chinese women?'

This judgemental attitude was in fact a reality, and we felt it. Many Chinese, especially those from privileged circumstances, such as those from the ranks of party Chinese, regarded us as people of a second-class order, subtypes of the human being, creatures who were tolerated because the government had ordered them to be here, and because their presence in China could be politically prestigious.

Again and again, the door of the clinic room opened and a woman's face appeared, trying to see what kind of a creature it was who had showed interest in them. It was the impudent German who had said he was up to espionage in Shanghai and who had gone on to say that he was out with a pretty Chinese girl. Evidently this was a fascinating escapade for these Chinese ladies, and they were tickled pink by the very idea.

Only Xiao Gu remained relentless. 'That is something the party clinic committee should deal with!'

Dr Kang, who in general was well inclined towards me, drew me aside during treatment and asked in English, 'Why are you doing this? Don't you feel happy with us? Aren't we doing enough to make you feel comfortable here?'

I shook my shoulders. I was not actually delighted with the situation, I had to admit.

'Tell me the truth, what actually took place yesterday evening in the town?'

'Oh, Dr Kang, you know full well how interesting Shanghai is at night. If you like, we can go out together and I'll show you its night life.'

'What!' As if electrified, Kang bristled and said in loud indignation, 'There's nothing of that kind in the city!'

'Oh yes,' I contradicted him, 'you just don't know about it, that's all. Come with Dr Haubensack and me one evening. We can take Xiao Gu with us. We'll show you both everything.'

Amused, he translated this to the speechless interpreter who, in the meantime, had turned deadly pale. She was so embarrassed by this offer that she rolled her eyes upwards, where they disappeared behind her thin upper lids.

'Oh, that I would never do!' she said. 'I stay at home in the evenings with my dictionaries and study.'

'That's not true,' I declared. 'How is it that you were busy observing me when I was at the tailor's and then later followed me for a bit on my way home, where you spied on me again?'

'Ugh?' she grunted. 'You are the one that's spying; you've admitted as much.'

In this way she tried to turn the tables against me. Dr Kang was very excited.

'No, Xiao Gu, you're the one that's doing the spying, Xiao Gui [little devil]!' said I.

'You have to tell me exactly what you were doing yesterday and what you were doing on the previous nights in Shanghai, Dr Ralf,' Kang demanded.

The first thing that occurred to me in answer to this was to tell them to go to hell, but then I felt that I had certain obligations with regard to my hosts, so I said, 'So that you all know the truth: in the evenings I sometimes go to the Seaman's Club near the Friendship Store, because there I can drink a beer in peace.'

'You shouldn't do that; you're not a seaman,' Kang said severely. 'The club is only for sailors and officers belonging to foreign ships anchored in the harbour.'

Oh, go to the devil, I wanted to say. This whole dirty spying business had become a pain in the neck. But Kang did a good job. He then went from room to room throughout the clinic and announced: 'Doctor Rompard is not involved in any kind of espionage. He just goes down to the Seaman's Club from time to time to enjoy a beer.' He came back to the clinic room pouring with sweat.

'And sometimes Dr Haubensack goes with me. He drinks a beer there, too,' I said to complete my account.

Kang ran off again immediately to proclaim to the staff that sometimes Dr Haubensack also went along to the Seaman's Club for a beer.

When he returned from his errand I said, 'If you come along with us, then there are three of us, you, Dr Haubensack and me, all three of us, and we can all drink a beer in the Seaman's Club together.' His eyes widened. 'Off you go, now,' I told him, 'and tell them all that we'll soon be a threesome in the club.'

But he did not set off for a third time. He grinned instead. Clearly, he could see the idiocy of it all. Privately, I thought to myself, 'My God, where will this general Chinese lunacy lead us? We have the feeling that this profound stupidity is not only a symptom rife among interpreters and doctors, but reaches up to the highest echelons of government.

That's the reason why the Chinese won't let us look into the cards, so to speak. It's simply because there's nothing to offer, and that goes for the highest positions in the state. Secretly, they themselves suspect how stupid they are! Consequently, they try their hardest to prevent foreigners from discovering just how backward and idiotic they are, so as not to be exposed. And, above all, the most important thing is not to lose face!

Politically Induced Stupidity

This modern Chinese 'stupidity' seems to me in the main to be politically induced. In the first place, Mao Tse-tung managed to get rid of the intelligentsia by either getting them to emigrate, throwing them in prison to rot or simply putting a bullet through their heads. After all this had been accomplished, there was only the brainless mass left over, a rabble which can be especially poisonous when it comes to power and influence. The mob cannot deal with these things; this we learned all too well in the Nazi period. In the same way that we children, along with the adults, were supposed to raise the right arm and endlessly repeat 'Heil Hitler' during the Nazi era, nowadays people in red China have to continuously echo the praise of their Great 'Helmsman', Mao Tse-tung. Mao's presence remains ubiquitous even after his death. Mao is still revered as the world's greatest statesman and politician; he's seen as the profound sage and philosopher, the most brilliant writer, the paramount scientist, an unfailing physician, the venerated prototype for each single Chinese person, etc. Everybody has to blare out Mao's praises all the time.

A reminiscence from the Nazi time came into my mind, and I related it to Achille.

When, as schoolboys, we went home after lessons we passed an animal shop with a beautiful parrot in front of its entrance ruffling his radiant green feathers. He tossed around on a little swing and greeted pedestrians with 'Heil Hitler'. The shopkeeper had taught him that as he wanted to attract more customers. We used to reply, 'Moin, moin,' the common Frisian greeting, when we stood before the shop, and the bird quickly repeated it. He recognised us from afar when we came, and shouted, 'Moin, moin – Heil Hitler!' Because the parrot was so teachable we taught him some more words. One of my chums used to say our most common word to him – namely, 'Arschloch [arsehole]' – and the parrot soon replied, 'Heil Hitler – Arschloch.'

The shopkeeper, a certain Herr Sengstake, was outraged and, of course, frightened when he heard his parrot vocalising such an indecent expression in connection with The Great Führer. He popped out of his shop and threatened us with a long stick whenever we came near. It was the early '40s and the newspapers were full of news about the war; the name of the British prime minister, Winston Churchill, was quite often mentioned, so everyone kept talking about Churchill, and when we again went by the shop one of us said casually, 'Churchill'. The parrot heard it and he echoed 'Churchill' straight away. He now used to say, 'Heil Hitler – moin, moin – Arschloch – Churchill' when he cheerfully opened his crooked beak and clawed around on his swing.

The proprietor hit the roof with fear and anger because some customers had become irritated with his heretical bird. He denounced us naughty boys to our headmaster, who felt scared as well and, in due turn, informed people in the Nazi Party. Two grim-looking SA fellows in yellow uniforms came into our classroom the next morning, and we four wrongdoers were told off in front of our classmates and then escorted by our teacher, the headmaster and the two grim-faced party men to the animal shop.

When the parrot saw our motley group coming along, he scented an unpleasant event and started screaming, 'Arschloch, Arschloch!' Our teacher was furious; he asked the shopman who had taught his parrot such evil words. 'That was your wicked pupils!' Herr Sengstake said. However, the two party men were amused. They laughed their heads off when they heard the bird shouting his swearwords, but our master slapped our faces.

The parrot continued, 'Churchill – Arschloch,' while he fixed his little round eyes at us and shouted this several times; the SA people seemed to be quite pleased.

'This bird is absolutely fabulous!' they said enthusiastically. 'He's quite a clever bird. Who taught him that?' We all four proudly pointed at our chests: 'We did. It was us!'

'Then you are very good Hitler boys,' one of the yellow men replied encouragingly.

We all calmed down now and the shopkeeper asked us in. We looked at his guinea pigs, rabbits, canary birds, turtles, goldfish and white mice. A big turtle had got a swastika painted on its back. One of the party members wanted to buy the turtle, but the shopkeeper gave it to him as a present.

'You'll just have to feed it with green salad leaves,' he instructed the new owner. 'What later comes out of its bottom looks yellowish, just like your uniform.'

The yellow watchman seemed a bit irritated by this and handed the turtle back to the shopkeeper, who said he should keep it because the turtle would bring good luck and a happy long life to its owner.

Outside, the parrot had started shouting again: 'Arschloch – Heil Hitler, Arschloch – Heil Hitler!'

Now the SA people began to seriously protest. 'This impudence is clearly violating the rules of the NSDAP, Herr Sengstake; the bird must be killed immediately!'

The shopkeeper was devastated. 'He's my only darling, you know,' he yammered. 'Since my wife passed away he is now my only close friend. If you want to murder him, you can kill me as well. Look how beautiful he is: he ruffles his shining green feathers, opens his hooked yellow beak and winks with his bright, intelligent eyes; he's a real marvel!'

The parrot screamed anxiously: 'Churchill – Arschloch, Churchill –

Arschloch.' He didn't stop shouting, so that it could be heard all over the street.

'And one can hear how intelligent my darling is,' the shopkeeper continued. 'He won't stop calling Churchill an arsehole. And that's bloody true!'

One of my buddies said: 'We taught him!'

'Very good, my lad,' the party man said, putting his hand on my friend's shoulder. 'Are you already members of our glorious Hitler Youth?'

'No,' we said, 'we're still too young.'

'Then I'll arrange it for you,' the yellow one said exuberantly. 'You'll all four become what we call "Underage Members of the Hitler Youth"!'

Both party men raised their right arm into the air and shouted in unison, 'Heil Hitler,' and the parrot answered them straight away with the identical words. One kept the turtle with the swastika under his arm as they left.

When the two chaps had marched off, they seemed to be quite content with what they had seen, heard and witnessed.

We were trotting back back to school accompanied by our teachers when we heard the parrot shouting again behind us: 'Heil Hitler – Arschloch, Heil Hitler – Arschloch.' The SA men had already got too far away to hear it. The headmaster punched us in the ribs. 'You wretched little bastards,' he hissed, 'that's what you are, all four of you! You'll be a nuisance in the Hitler Youth, and you know it!' We kept our mouths shut.

When the war had come to an end our school was completely burnt out and we enjoyed long holidays lasting the whole summer and autumn of 1945. One day, I wanted to see whether the animal shop still existed and whether the parrot had survived. The shopkeeper stood in front of his door, recognised me at once and looked quite happy when he saw me.

'Where is your parrot?' I asked.

'Oh yes, my boy, nice to see you. I'll tell you. He brought me lots of luck, I'll tell you, my friend.' And then he recounted what had happened.

One day in May an English soldier had stepped into his shop. He heard the parrot scream, 'Heil Hitler!' The shopkeeper had strictly kept the bird in the cellar after the armistice, because it constantly shouted the words it had learned.

'Are you hiding a Nazi gangster somewhere on your premises?' the soldier asked suspiciously.

'He's my parrot,' the shame-faced shopman replied.

'Then he has to be removed, mister,' the Englishman said firmly. 'I'm awfully sorry, but it's against the rules of the military authorities. This parrot must be put down.'

'No,' the shopkeeper answered. 'He's all I've got, and he's my only darling!'

'You have the cheek to say that?' the Briton replied accusingly. 'I'll report you to my colonel and tell him about you and your bird!' The soldier went away.

The next afternoon, an officer in an earth-brown uniform came in carrying a long cane which he swirled around in the air. He wanted to see the parrot, was quite friendly and seemed be pleasantly amused when he heard what the bird had to say. The downcast shopman let him listen to the parrot's entire repertoire: 'Heil Hitler – moin, moin – Arschloch – Churchill.'

'What an extremely intelligent bird you've got there,' the colonel marvelled. 'I'd like to buy him!'

Herr Sengstake was flabbergasted. 'You want to buy him?'

'Yes. Please give him to me. You know, I could easily seize him from you and have him put to sleep because of his suspicious vocabulary. But that's not our English way.'

The shopkeeper was a shrewd businessman.

'He's my only darling,' he moaned. 'Since my wife died he's all I've got.'

'Please, do let me have this wonderful bird,' the officer said persuasively.

'You won't put him down then?'

'Oh no! I'll take him home and show him to my folks to make them laugh and let them see what idiots Nazi parrots were. We'll have great fun together, including the parrot.'

'Moin, moin,' cried the bird.

'OK,' said the shopkeeper (he had adopted this phrase as the first words learned from the victorious foreigners), 'OK, sir, you can have him for, er, one thousand pounds.'

Sengstake took paper and a pen and clearly wrote in numbers and letters, 'One 1.000 £ Sterling'. He had learned some English in his younger days.

'One thousand pounds? That's an awful lot of money,' the Englishman sighed.

'You won't find a parrot like this in the whole world,' the animal seller explained. And now the officer started bargaining.

'Let's say 600 pounds,' he suggested vaguely.

The parrot twisted his head into a slanted position and scornfully watched the two men bartering about his value. He seemed to sense what was going on and shouted 'Arschloch, Arschloch!'

'How wonderful,' the colonel enthusiastically remarked.

Sengstake said: '900 pounds.'

The parrot screamed, 'Churchill – Churchill!'

'No, 700.'

'Not less than 800 pounds, sir! It'll break my heart anyway. But just for you, sir, because you're an English gentleman, I'll sell him to you for 800 pounds.'

'Heil Hitler,' the bird affirmed, ruffling his feathers.

'It's a deal,' the colonel consented. 'I'll bring you the money tomorrow and will collect my parrot then. I'd like to teach him some ugly words to add to his remarkable list!' And that's what happened.

On the black market the shopkeeper changed the sterling money he had received from the colonel into Reichsmarks. It was a great amount of almost worthless German cash. But he could now refurbish his shop which had been badly damaged by shells and bombs, and he stocked it with new white rabbits, hamsters, turtles, guinea pigs, goldfish, plus a beautiful young parrot whom he taught 'Moin, moin' first and then 'How do you do!', which was the longest phrase a parrot ever had to learn from him.

Meanwhile, the colonel spread the gospel about this Heil-Hitler-shouting parrot among his fellow soldiers and every day the animal shop was full of British servicemen who all asked for another such a parrot who could say 'Heil Hitler'. But the only one who could say as much had gone with the colonel, and the animal merchant didn't have the courage to teach his new parrot the taboo words. The shopkeeper had a lot to do anyway painting swastikas on the back of countless turtles which he had already sold at handsome prices to members of the occupying forces.

One day in July, an American general came over from Bremen. He introduced himself as Brigadier General McPherson. His British fellow officer, the colonel, had told him about the wonderful parrot which he had bought in the animal shop. Escorted by two GIs, the American stormed through the door, banged on the counter table with his large hairy fist several times and demanded a Heil-Hitler-shouting parrot on the spot!

The shopkeeper humbly apologised, saying that these two words were prohibited now and absolutely banned after the Nazi period – thank God! – had ended. But the Yankee remained adamant. In the meatime his GIs were busy champing their gum.

'Man!' the officer roared, 'I'll pay you one thousand US dollars in cash for such a bird!

The shopkeeper shuddered.

'And if you don't want to cooperate I'll close your shop down and have you sentenced by a military court for possessing such a fascist animal at all, and you'll spend some time in jail.' He hammered his plump, porcupine-like fists on the table to the rhythm of his speech in order to make his dictum sound more impressive. 'Do you want that, eh?'

A quiver ran down the shopkeeper's spine. He trembled all over as he promised to teach his new parrot 'Heil Hitler' as soon as he could.

The officer thundered: 'I'll be back, next week, same day, same hour, my German friend. Keep that in mind.' Then he tramped out with his two escorts, slamming the shop door behind him.

That very evening the animal seller cautiously locked himself up with his young parrot in one of the garret rooms and started teaching him 'Heil Hitler'. He repeated this lesson every night, and after five nights the bird could clearly say the spooky words without difficulty. Thus instructed, however, the parrot had to be kept in a soundproof place until the American general showed up again to take him. Herr Sengstake even closed the bird's mouth by wrapping adhesive plaster tightly around his yellow beak and only taking it off to feed him. The shopman was still frightened and made absolutely sure that not one of his neighbours could hear the bird's repetitions, something that could have happened any time, as they would then have called the police – meaning, in those days, military police – and Herr Sengstake would have been in great trouble.

To cut a long story short, the general bought the parrot for a thousand US dollars. During the summer and autumn months of 1945 a whole army of British and American soldiers flocked into the merchant's shop. They all wanted to buy a parrot who could shout 'Heil Hitler'. The shopkeeper acquired one parrot after the other and taught them all to say the forbidden words. When there was a sudden shortage of parrots in Germany, the colonel, who kept visiting Herr Sengstake's shop, assisted him in getting a number of beautiful parrots from England, because the demand was just so great. A whimsical English civil servant had read Hitler's *Mein Kampf* and wanted to buy a parrot who could shout, 'Ein Volk, ein Reich, ein Fuehrer!', but this turned out to be too long a phrase for an ordinary parrot to remember. So he had to make do with a phrase of the more humdrum kind.

By the end of the summer, the shopkeeper had sold some hundreds of parrots who could all shout 'Heil Hitler' to members of the occupation army, and he had received one thousand dollars from American buyers or eight hundred pounds sterling from British customers for each single bird, not to mention the swastika-garnished turtles which sold over the counter like hotcakes for mere peanuts. Herr Sengstake had made roughly one hundred thousand US dollars in a few months and became one of the richest people in our town after the war. He was the first wealthy person after the horrible Nazis had gone, and he had become so with the miraculous help of some feather-ruffling parrots who could shout scandalous phrases. The shopkeeper was clever enough to buy a number of ruined sites and bombed-out houses; he acquired real estate and wasteland, and after a short while he could afford to retire. But as far as I know, he always kept a parrot until, in the '60s, he, then in his late eighties, died. Whether these birds were still able to shout 'Heil Hitler' is not known.

When I had ended my story Achille said, 'That's something like the "east wind prevailing over the west wind", as Mao Tse-tung once said in a speech addressed to Russian students in Moscow.'

'I would say it's something like the "Unity of the Opposites",' I mused, 'which is another of Mao's common phrases, but can, however, be traced back to the beginnings of human reasoning and thought in the East and the West.'

The state of affairs in China could not but remind me of Nazi times in Germany. In those days, too, there was enormous political pressure, which we adolescents experienced at that time as a painful curtailment of our freedom. The empty, stereotyped political slogans dribbled out each day here in China by party imbeciles forcibly recalled for me those hated days spent serving in the Hitler Youth movement. This requirement to serve was foisted on us all, and there was nothing of interest in it other than to watch how stupid people could be in maintaining what they considered to be an emergency situation. Exactly the same was true for the situation here, and it must have been true for the German Democratic Republic created after the war, I imagined, as I remembered passing through the eastern sector of Berlin. On those occasions, West Berlin folks would have been subjected to the futile indignities of long waits for their baggage to be checked and for passport control, and would have been ordered to get out of the cross-border train, then having to wait on windy platforms while they were forced to go through several other forms of petty harassment.

Later, it was the same on car journeys from West to East Berlin. The checks began with the tearing off of hubcaps, followed by the inspection of the under parts of the car with a torch and mirror as though we in the West had nothing better to do than spy on our spiritually impoverished neighbour. I hate all totalitarian regimes for these restrictions of human freedom, but above all for the way in which they are the vehicles for supporting and promoting human stupidity.

At least as far as I was concerned, this period of study in China didn't so much serve the function of helping me to come to know more about Chinese methods of healing as it acquainted me as a medical professional from the West with the hideous outrages of a fully organised police state at close quarters. In fact, the whole horror could not have represented a better plea in favour of our democratic society.

Then, something interesting happened. A letter arrived for Alice after fourteen days' delay, during which it had evidently been opened, and on its envelope someone had written something by hand in Chinese. Words had been struck out and corrected. The message was:

'The party controls everything, but who controls the party?'

Alice took the letter to old Mr Lu, who translated the Chinese for her. At the same time, she protested that the letter had taken such a long time to arrive and that it had been opened. Lu promised to look into the matter.

This trivial incident showed that there is perhaps something of a secret opposition to China abroad, and in this case it made use of the opportunity to smuggle out opinion against the dominant political administration. Apparently, in this way it can show the party organisation that it cannot control everything.

Achille had fallen into conversation with the warrior's son, Balu, from Cameroon. Balu was fully convinced that in Europe there are a hundred million unemployed, that all workers have to go hungry, that when they fall ill, they receive no medical attention, and that, as a consequence, they die off like flies from epidemics. Further, he believed that living conditions in Europe are worse than those prevailing in the People's Republic of China. The people in Europe are not free either, not like the Chinese are here. According to Balu, they are conditioned and eaten up by capitalism, whereas the Chinese in their present communist society are really free.

'Why did you want to adopt Ralf's religion, then, Balu?' Achille asked him. 'A religion only enslaves you.'

'Ah, well, you know,' Balu explained, 'it wasn't the religion so much as that beautiful new Mercedes.'

It was strange to hear such a false assessment from an African academic, a warrior's son and a doctor to boot. Perhaps that's the way black Africa sees us from its perspective.

Yesterday evening, the interpreter Fishface came along after we had bought things from the Friendship Store. We named him such as he was extremely skinny, he had an emaciated bony, scaly face and a deeply wrinkled forehead topped with gluey pomaded grey hair on his skull, and he wore huge thick eye-glasses which made him look like a fish. Recently, he had become my personal 'protector' and was appointed by the party as a watchdog, ever since my faux pas as an alleged 'spy'. We chatted with each other for a while.

'Well, now, you've seen a lot of things at our place by now, two months in

China, that's quite something. You've learned all about Chinese medicine; you've deepened the friendship between our two countries . . .'

I interrupted him. 'Do you really think we've learned much about Chinese medicine?'

Fishface was much taken aback. 'Well, of course! That's what our professors and doctors have been showing you all the time!'

'Do you really believe that that's Chinese medicine?'

His face turned to stone. 'Well, we're here in China, what else could it be?' he stuttered.

'Today's China is not the real China,' I said simply.

'What else could it be?' Fishface asked.

'It's a European province, an appalling and terrifying caricature, an imitation of an oddly perverted communist Europe which, thank God, doesn't exist. It's something that has nothing to do with either European tradition or Chinese, no, not in the least.'

Fishface wheezed. It was clear that he wanted to get at what I meant.

'What more can we do for you?' he asked weakly.

'You have to send your Chinese doctors into the world, let them go to Europe so that they can see for themselves what's really going on and how modern medicine is run. Your folks have not the slightest idea about Europe. Let your doctors and your academics travel. What they need is a real scientific and cultural exchange, but that situation is far, far away.'

He remained silent. He was horrified at what he had heard. 'Yes, well, when we've finished building up our socialism, then we can start talking about such things, but not at the moment,' he said.

Achilles and I then asked him whether he could travel where and when he wanted to, and he replied that of course when the party ordered him to, 'I can go where I like!'

'And who determines where and when?' Achille enquired.

'The party, of course,' said Fishface.

'And if you personally want to go off without the party's specific permission, what then?'

'Well, then I can't go,' Fishface replied, somewhat downcast.

'You see,' Achille pursued, 'it's different with us. We can travel whenever we like and wherever we like. I'm a free Frenchman; I can leave my country at any time and go somewhere else if I want to – and Dr Rompard can do the same.'

Fishface armed himself against possible attack. 'But then you have to ask the other states whether you may visit them or not?'

'No,' Achille replied, 'that's just it. In Europe anyone can travel wherever he wants to and whenever he wants to; we can even travel to America if necessary and don't even need a visa.'

This simply amazed Fishface. He asked me whether what Haubensack had said was true, and I confirmed that it was.

'We hear things about Europe, the West and its inhabitants which are quite different from what you've just mentioned,' he said doubtfully.

'Those things are not true,' we said together. 'Here, you have to listen to lies every day.'

Fishface was out for the count. We broke off proceedings there and then.

From there, we went back again into the Friendship Store, but this time we used another bridge that was a little removed from our usual path, because the hundred-year-old iron construction built by the British that we were in the habit of using was currently under repair. We needed quite a bit of time to try on the new suits and to converse with the tailor. On our way, we met Herr Gröber. He said that just at the moment it was awful here; one met no one and so there was hardly any occasion for a sensible conversation. So we suggested that we all go to the Seaman's Club for a cool drink, and perhaps schnapps into the bargain.

He then told us that he had been commissioned to write an article for a West German Socialist Democratic Party periodical on the intellectual climate here in Shanghai. He told us that he wanted to write honestly and mention that intellectuals here live in an atmosphere of fear and repression, that the events of the 'Cultural Revolution' have not been forgotten, and that intellectuals are shorn of all freedom and potential. He was convinced that such an article would never see the light of day in Germany, because it would tell the truth about today's circumstances in mainland China. In East Germany, they only wanted to hear lies about the country and the socialist paradise.

'We have to tell the truth to the free world, since nobody in Europe knows the truth of what's going on here,' Achille said. 'There, they worship an ignorant view of Chinese medicine, and labour under the illusion that this country is a paradise for the worker. They believe the rubbish that is spread throughout the world by its cunning communist propaganda, whereas in reality, folks here have to put up with hell!'

We sipped thoughtfully at our beer.

Chinese Womanly Curiosity

When we had all returned from the clinic and met each other again for the evening meal, Adrienne Coningk pulled at my arm and asked whether we could have a talk after dinner about something confidential. I said that it would be most comfortable upstairs in our apartment, but she said that wouldn't be suitable as she really had to talk to me in utmost confidence. Achille was not to know of anything; she felt that he was too cynical and coarse. So we sat down in a room next to the restaurant.

'You have some experience in buying books here,' she began.

'Yes, one has to know a bit of Chinese, and then it's really simple. What would you like to buy then?'

'Hmm, I find myself in a strange position; actually, it's something to laugh about.'

'Let me share your laugh. What books do you want?'

'I need an anatomical atlas with pictures.'

'In Chinese?'

'In Chinese.'

'Why?'

'Listen. And this must remain something strictly between us. Yesterday evening, the two interpreters came by, Xiao Han and Xiao Wang. They wanted to talk to Alice and me in our room. I was surprised. We spoke about this and that and how different the Europeans are from Chinese, and then Wang asked whether European women looked the same as Chinese. Alice and I laughed out loud, because we thought it was a pretty daft question. They knew, of course, they said, that we had a different facial structure, that much was clear, and that their Chinese eyes were formed, as we say in French, like an almond. Chinese women had a different hair colour and their eyebrows were much thicker, and they are usually smaller built than European women.

' "Yes, we know all that of course," said I.

'Xiao Han fluted, "We find European women really beautiful, much more so than Chinese."

'In answer to this, we said we were flattered to hear that, but they must remember that there are lovely Chinese women, too. Both of them were good examples. The interpreters giggled.

' "We don't mean that, though," they giggled again, "we want to know whether European women are the same 'below' as Chinese women, or are there any differences, for example?"

' "Below?" Alice asked, dumbfounded. "What do you mean?"

'Xiao Han opened her legs and pointed to her crotch with her finger and made a quick movement from back to front along her dark blue Mao slacks.

' "That there, between your legs," Xiao Han said, and Xiao Wang nodded in eager confirmation.

' "What should we have down there? We look exactly like Chinese women," we both said, not without some embarrassment.

' "We'd like to know for sure," the two interpreters blurted.

' "I'd not expected anything like that," I said.'

I was astonished. 'In a word, Ralf,' Adrienne continued, 'they asked us to show them our genitals, and for this privilege, they wanted to show us theirs. We were shocked, I can tell you, and of course we declined.'

'I would not have thought that possible, considering how prudish they are in general,' I said. I could not help but shake my head in astonishment. Then I laughed at the very idea.

'And then?' I asked.

'Well, I want to show them with the help of a book on anatomy just what European and Chinese women look like "down there" – in other words, assure them that we're the same.'

'That's a good idea,' I said. 'When do you need the book? You can come with me into the bookstore if you like, Adrienne.'

'You could find the very thing I need on your own, I'm sure, Ralf,' Adrienne replied.

'I find this story amusing,' I said. 'Do you think I could relate it to Achille?'

'Well, if you want to,' the Dutchwoman said, 'but you know what he's like. He'll immediately make a dirty joke out of the whole thing and even go so far as to tell the other colleagues, interpreters and cadre members. I definitely don't want that to happen. I have no wish to expose these two. Achille has to swear that he'll keep the matter to himself. Otherwise everyone will lose face.'

I cycled to the college in the afternoon and on the way back stopped at the large bookstore in Nanjing Road. The booksellers already knew me there. I went over to the medical shelves and discovered something suitable. It was a thick, newly published edition with a green dust cover entitled *Textbook of Anatomy of the Human Body*. It was printed on the cheapest paper, but had good black-and-white illustrations. I thumbed through it. Yes, there was a picture showing the female genitalia. That was the right book. It cost 5 yuan, the equivalent of 3 euros.

At the cash desk, the bookseller wanted to know why I needed this particular book. I showed him my swimming-card ID which made it clear that I was employed at a medical clinic and institute in Shanghai. That was enough for him.

Once back at the hotel, I showed Achille my purchase and told him the spicy story of the two women.

'There, you see what really interests Chinese women?' he said. 'They're mainly interested in sex! And it's forbidden here, although everyone's interested in it, everybody thinks about it. They should show their pretty Chinese genitalia to us European men. But they dare not, because of their wretched party. So they turn to European women!'

Achille was very keen to see the pictures of female genitalia as illustrated in the newly purchased Chinese volume.

'Aha!' he said. 'That looks great – but everything's in Chinese, dammit!'

'The Latin term is in brackets behind it.'

'Can these Chinese correctly give the anatomical names for the illustrations in Chinese?'

'They can do that very well. The Chinese have simply taken over our Latin terms precisely and introduced them into their own language. Latin can lead occasionally to misunderstanding. A German sinologist, for example, once bluntly translated the concepts of Chinese medicine into the Latin of the kitchen, in the hope that it would sound a little more scientific. But what then finally issued from this questionable translation was simply so much gobbledegook.'

The next day, I showed the anatomical book to Adrienne. She thought it was a very good idea to use it to demonstrate to the two Chinese interpreters, and asked me to lend her the book for a few days, which I did.

'What did they say?' I asked Adrienne when I met her again the other day.

'They had come to our room again, and they simply laughed at the book,' she told me. ' "No, we want to see your fanny in full!" they demanded. What could we do? They had already quickly got out of their clothes.

'Alice was the first to strip off after the two Chinese women had got undressed. I could not avoid having to do the same as them. Xiao Han and Xiao Wang were sitting at the bedside, having opened their thighs for us to look at their intimate parts. When we showed them ours they seemed to be disappointed. "Oh, you look pretty much the same like us," Xiao Wang said, surprised. "We've always assumed European women had much more spectacular intimate parts than us."

' "What's the reason, then, for European men getting so extremely thrilled about women?" Xiao Han asked, and kept shaking her head in disillusionment.

' "I really don't know the answer," said I, and Alice agreed.

'They seemed to be extremely disappointed when they discovered that we looked pretty much the same "there below" as them.

'"It is completely different from what we've been told," Xiao Wang said.

'"What were you told then?"

'"That European women have incredibly exciting vaginas, turning western men on to make love with them like mad."

'"It's all nonsense," we said. And the two women went off as quickly as they had come.'

When Adrienne told me this episode it made me laugh again, and she soon joined in so we both laughed for quite a while.

'Please don't tell Achille,' she pleaded, and I promised her I wouldn't.

The Complicated Business of Sending a Parcel

Yesterday, I packed a number of books into six parcels and took them to the post office. I was obliged to open these at the counter, however, and several post office officials took turns at thrusting their dirty fingers between the pages and generally rummaging around, and in so doing, threw everything into disorder. It had taken me hours of work to regulate and classify the material. They told me that I would not be allowed to send off a text in French which the College of Chinese Medicine had issued as official teaching material, since it may well contain certain secrets. If I really wanted to post it, I would first have to produce a written explanation for the post office, stamped with the college seal, which would prove that I had received official permission to send this book concerning instructions for the practice of acupuncture – that was, in my opinion, very poorly printed and on a very cheap kind of paper – to Europe.

'Why do you think I've come here at all?' I asked the unfriendly man at the reception desk.

What could he say to this? He remained silent.

'My government has sent me here in order to study Chinese medicine and acupuncture, and now you tell me that I can't even send my teaching material back home with me!'

I had the impression that I'd wasted my time in China. After all, over three months had passed since I'd first arrived in the country, and it seemed to me now that this had been lost time. *Lost Time Spent in China* – that could be the title of a book, but who would believe me? Everybody in the West wants to hear more about the Chinese 'miracle' of acupuncture – that is, hear something good about it, something positive and constructive – but the acupuncture I had experienced here was a mere castle in the air, a medical phantom born of Chinese frustration.

The man in front of me either did not understand or did not want to understand. He muttered something to himself which sounded like: 'Everything that concerns Chinese medicine is a strictly safeguarded official state secret. And even in the case where a European has studied medicine here, upon leaving the country he should promptly forget all that he has learned.'

The official removed the string with which the parcels were tied and refused to give it back to me. Happily for me, Fishface appeared at that moment with a letter to post. I asked him for help, and he explained in no uncertain terms to the custodians of official regulation that the string for these parcels had been correctly purchased by me, and was therefore my property.

At this, one of the employees disappeared into a back room and after a full ten minutes reappeared with a frayed and spliced ball of string of the poorest quality. I protested that this was not my ball of string, at which those behind the counter maintained as one man that I was not telling the truth. Fishface once more jumped into the fray, insisting that in all Shanghai there was not a ball of string of this contemptible quality to be bought and that it must certainly have originated in some capitalistic country abroad. He said that he knew exactly what my string looked like, since he had been present when I bought the said ball of string (which wasn't true).

Again, one of the employees vanished for another quarter of an hour and returned at last with the ball of string that I had bought myself. Fishface and I tied up the parcels once more, and all six parcels had to be weighed a second time. It turned out during this procedure that one of the parcels was heavier than the permitted 500 grams. It was not permitted to send parcels out of the country that were heavier than 500 grams, declared the man at the parcels service who, up to now, had been standing silently in the background with a miserable expression on his face. In compliance with this, we accordingly untied the offending parcel, removed two of the books it contained and tied it up again, and only then were we able to finally pay the required postage and actually hand the things over for forwarding. I was exhausted by all this and bathed in sweat. Outside and inside, the temperature stood at 37°C. On top of this, it was very humid, and there was not a piece of air-conditioning apparatus to be seen anywhere. The whole transaction had lasted two and a half hours. Not only was my midday break well over by that time, but I was also long overdue for lunch. It was probable that there was already somebody looking for me in the hotel or at the clinic.

Fishface kindly promised to take care of things for me, and also arranged a special vehicle to get me to the clinic. Although grateful for this, I still had to go to the hotel for a shower and change of clothes. I could not think of treating patients in this condition, exhausted and sweated through as I was.

Quite apart from the heat and the stifling air in the post office, what annoyed me most was the unparalleled bloody-mindedness and curiosity of these post office officials. Before the appearance of Fishface, for example, these public servants had asked me all kinds of questions that had nothing whatsoever to do with sending the parcels.

The whole affair was akin to a police interrogation, but what could I do? It was impossible to fly back with so many books in addition to my personal baggage. I was therefore left with the alternatives of either sending them home by post or leaving them here in China.

I began to think about what the supervisor at the post office had said about Chinese medicine being a political state secret. If this was really the case, why had they allowed western doctors into the country at all? What was the point of all the wearisome preparation on the part of the German Ministry of Health to make this stay possible, or the official reception at the German embassy in Beijing or that at the Chinese Ministry of Health? Why the boring political claptrap at the welcoming ceremony on our arrival, as well as at the college and at every little institute we had visited? Why was all this thought to be necessary? Gradually, it dawned on me that in reality there was no great interest in acquainting us with the techniques of acupuncture and needle analgesia, and that there was no real intention on the part of the Chinese Communist Party to initiate us into the scientific authenticity of Chinese methods of healing. So what actually was the intention? I would eventually find out what it was.

On the way back to the hotel, Fishface explained to me that, as a member of the Chinese Communist Party, he was enabled to put a certain amount of pressure on civil servants. I told him quite plainly that the chicanery that I'd been subjected to by public authorities was frankly disgraceful. I showed him the text that we had studied and worked on for three months every day, and complained about the fact that we were not even allowed to take it out of the country. This, I said, was an example of China's incredible backwardness. In reply, he merely referred to the political regulations within China, and said that there was nothing folks could do about it. He didn't like this kind of thing either.

'Then why don't you rise up against these stupid regulations?' I asked.

He replied to the effect that these were simply the party's regulations and that one had to abide by them. For him, it seemed to be the most natural thing in the world. That was how it was here; people in China didn't even dare to think about objecting to the palpable idiocy of party laws. They were so thoroughly brainwashed and lived under such enormous psychological pressure that they were no longer able to think for themselves or utter a personal opinion. In reply to this, I said that surely there were some sensible Chinese who could enquire for themselves as to why these imbecile regulations were there at all, and whether they could be replaced by better, more intelligent ordinances.

As a reaction to my indignation, Fishface laughed his curious laugh, which sounded like the protests of a shooed-away hen.

'Is it because the party is afraid, perhaps, that secret information could leak abroad?' I asked.

He grinned and his shortsighted eyes peered at me through his thick lenses. 'Yes,' he said after a moment's reflection, 'that could very well be the case.'

'As an emissary of my government, I would very much like to enquire somewhere why there are such loony rules here in the People's Republic. But where can one make such enquiries? In Europe, such a thing is possible at any time. For example, I can write at any time to the chancellor, to the head of state, to the president of the state I reside in, to my respective member of parliament or to a federal representative. I would then receive an answer to my enquiry. But who's responsible here for that kind of thing? The party perhaps? As a party member yourself, you should know all about it.'

He said that I could not find an answer to my question unless I were to enquire at the embassy in Beijing. I decided there and then that that is what I would do. I would complain to my ambassador there. But what would he say? His answer would probably go like this:

'Dr Rompard, you are aware of course of the fact that you have come to a totalitarian state and that's how things are here. Things are not easy for us diplomats either. What you have to report is something that our embassy people have to put up with every day. We try to accommodate ourselves to the situation, you see. Now why don't you do the same thing?'

I have to add that Fishface during the whole of this time, in the post office as well as on the way home, exhibited both great patience and willingness to help.

On our way back to the hotel Fishface asked me, 'Have you ever seen Mao Tse-tung in person?'

'No, how could I?'

'You visited China three years ago when Mao was still alive.'

'There was no opportunity then to see him. Have you ever seen Mao yourself?'

'Yes, I have,' he replied.

'When and where?'

'It was twelve years ago at a party meeting in Beijing.'

Fishface's small eyes flashed through his thick goggles.

'And how was it?'

He cleared his throat noisily. 'Mao looked unbelievably beautiful!'

'Tell me!'

'His full face was rosy and young, his bushy, well-groomed black hair was shining, his lips were red like our Chinese national colours, I could clearly see the wart on his chin. I still view him like this, even after so many years!'

'That sounds amazing!'

'It was! I saw people fainting when they came close to him, especially a number of women among them. We attendants were all under a rapturous spell.' At this point Fishface seemed to realise that he had verbalised something which was not quite in line with the official regulations; he giggled in a high voice as he added with an apology: 'Anyway, my knees went weak, they just gave way and I was trembling all over.'

Back at the apartment I told Achille about Fishface's revelation. My colleague laughed and said in contempt, 'That's just as mad as these girlish fans at a pop concert of the Beatles, or like the Roman Catholic believers on Saint Peter's Square in Rome when they look up to their pontiff. The people and the rulers seem to fit nicely together,' he remarked drily. 'They completely fulfil each other's needs.'

Achille and I then talked about China's attempt to reach the same technical standard as the West. At this particular moment, the Chinese were experiencing a situation whereby their old, indigenous culture was apparently in its last throes. Much of China's tradition had been castigated as backward, and condemned or simply forbidden. On the other hand, much of what had been imported from the West, such as the washing machine, the car, television and other technical advances, was admired, but these things had been by no means as perfected as they were in our own society. A good example of what I mean here can be found in the practice of western medicine in such spheres as surgery, the regulation of medical prescriptions and the application of medical technology. We saw this in the example of the ancient X-ray apparatus dating back to 1925, and in the case of inadequate examinations of the eye and the ear. In the hands of the Chinese, western technologies were reduced to mere caricatures of the original procedures.

It was a pleasant Sunday morning, and at 7.30 a.m. I was already standing in front of the hotel. Screeching female voices with their revolutionary songs and unnatural, mechanical tremolos had been screaming from innumerable loudspeakers since 5 a.m. Between these ballads, one heard the howling of the two-stringed erhu, the Chinese knee violin, playing a heart-rending melody, and all this amid the hooting of cars and lorries and the chattering engines of motorboats on the river. The hooter is the most important accessory for a Chinese driver. It is not used as a short signal as with us, but is applied in a prolonged blast and aggressively at least four or five times, so that it is noticed, and so effectively gets on the nerves. This ceaseless acoustic pressure had blunted our hearing and made every kind of intellectual activity impossible. It was all part of the consciously applied red Chinese machinery, calculated to render everyone an imbecile, as none of it can be satisfactorily processed by the human brain.

In the evening, we all sat in the bar together. With us was a Yugoslavian seaman serving on the German merchant ship the *Bieberstein*, which plied between Hamburg and Shanghai on the Hapag-Lloyd line. He had finally gone on land to fly back home. He told us that security personnel at the hotel had recorded a conversation today between him and his wife. He had heard his own voice on tape coming from the telephone switchboard room. It was an exact recording of what he had said to his wife a few hours before. When he asked the porter why his voice was to be heard issuing from that direction on tape, he was firmly told that this was not his voice, but that of someone else. Why, then, had this person spoken in his own tongue, the seaman enquired? The laconic reply was that modern China was simply an international state.

As a citizen of another communist state, he complained bitterly about being subjected to this kind of outrageous indignity; it was simply beneath the belt, and therefore disgusting. We told him that we too were constantly being bugged and that our letters were opened and scrutinised, and that, further, we were spied upon round the clock. We had gradually become used to it.

'You'd best get away from here as soon as possible!' he cried.

Achille is Arrested

Yesterday afternoon, Haubensack had made a three-hour city walking tour of the neighbouring district and had taken photos to record the experience. While doing so, he was arrested by soldiers of the People's Army, despite the fact that he had worn his nice green Chinese military uniform. He was carted off to a local street committee, where he was asked to produce his 'swim identification card'. This ID card officially certified that he was employed at the College of Chinese Medicine in Shanghai. This helped him, and after he submitted it, the people on the committee were friendlier. Achille courteously removed his military cap and told his jailers very convincingly that he was a friend of China, and that, formerly, he had been a member of the Communist Party in France which, probably because of his Red Army apparel, they immediately believed. Delighted, they all lined up to be photographed by him in front of the door of the decayed hut to which they had brought him.

Back at the hotel, he winked at me and said, 'With this hat in your hand, you can get through any land – including China!' How right he was.

In passing, as a matter of interest, there seemed to be special privileges for highly placed party members. One of the interpreters told me, for example, that in the hospital where we practised our acupuncture, there was a very well-appointed department for senior party functionaries. I then asked her how it was that in a country like China where, as everyone knew, there were no social distinctions, certain party members were entitled to special concessions. Was modern communist China in fact a class society?

For a moment, this question was an embarrassment as she realised that she had opened her mouth too wide, and then she tried to correct matters.

'Yes,' she added, 'before the Cultural Revolution, such concessions were possible, but today things are different.'

The infamous Gang of Four, she went on, had sought to introduce such privileges for senior officials, but all that was in the past. However, I noticed that she was very put off by my manner, since I had noticed that she wanted to lie to me. There was no doubt about the fact that senior functionaries still enjoyed great prerogatives, and did not wish to be placed on the same level as ordinary folk. Mr Gröber had already mentioned that the offspring of these people would often talk in the students' hostel of the super apartments they occupied in Beijing, apartments furnished and equipped with every creature comfort, with several bathrooms, TV sets, washing machines and refrigerators.

Once again, we had a routine day at the clinic behind us and didn't exactly know what to do with our time in the evening. Every contact with the Chinese was systematically squashed, and as a result we sat around and were both in a bad mood. Out of sheer boredom, we cursed China and the Chinese and asked ourselves how on earth doctors could practise good medicine at all under such appalling living conditions. If, when we returned to Europe, we came back with generally negative impressions of the country, then it was the Chinese who were to blame. The clumsy psychological treatment we experienced here seemed to demonstrate a tendency to reject rather than support the ostensible advancements claimed for communist China. Each day that passed registered a loss of income for our surgeries in Europe because we could not be there to work in them and here we were instead, cooped up like slaves. I tried to bring some consolation into the matter by reminding Achille and myself of the fact that the situation was much worse for simple people and for our professional colleagues.

A Good Restaurant in Shanghai

This afternoon, Herr Gröber and I went out to buy a few books. We talked about our European attitudes towards the Chinese and that of the Chinese towards us. They are indeed different from us, we agreed, but they can be very friendly and pleasant on occasion, and this we have to take into account. We became aware of this whenever we unexpectedly came across ordinary people in the street and knew that we were not being observed.

After making our purchases, we found ourselves in a Cantonese restaurant in Nanjing Road and were not shown into a separate room, but instead ate with all the other guests. Looking round, I noticed that at one time the place must have been an elegant restaurant. The service was good. However, at the end of the meal, we were presented with an enormous bill, apparently one that had been appropriately blown up for foreigners. There was the general conviction here that all westerners were millionaires. Gröber explained to the waiter that he should not mistake us for western capitalists, for such we certainly were not, but ordinary students who were in China to learn about things that would add to China's distinction and so spread its international esteem throughout the world. However, the waiter was not to be duped by this, and immediately explained that what we had eaten was much better quality than that presented to the average Chinese. We had to admit that the meal was excellent and footed the bill without further ado.

On the way back, we talked about the fact that there were still traces of the old culture to be seen here and there, vestiges which went unnoticed and unacknowledged by day tourists and travellers who only stopped for a short while. The ancient art of painting and calligraphy was one of these. The Chinese calligrapher meditates for a long time before putting his brush to paper. This aspect is reflected in the characters; there is something special and unique in the way the strokes are composed. According to ancient tradition, this, too, is how medicine should be practised. One should take plenty of time to talk to the patient, look carefully at his face and tongue, note the timbre of his voice, thoroughly enquire into his medical history, feel his pulse over a long period (at least for a hundred beats), take time in selecting the needle foramina (passages) in the case of acupuncture and, for certain needle therapies, carefully choose and prescribe the appropriate herbs in an atmosphere of peace and calm. In the hustle and bustle of life in the average clinic, little of this is possible. Everything must be managed quickly, since there are usually dozens of other patients waiting outside for treatment. It is not so very different in the typical German general practitioner's surgery. All appears to be standardised and worked out, but that is not the correct classic Chinese approach.

The meditation practised by the calligrapher may not be very different from that in Zen, and it points up the high quality of the configurations he draws. It is the same in the art of healing, whereby the good Chinese doctor will bring a certain meditative attitude to his work. This composure, though, has been displaced today by a brutal party political order imposed on the clinics of the country, favouring a mechanical sequence of events and mindless standardisation. Mindlessness – that is a widespread evil in this land. Who could ever think independently under such unrelenting pressure? Moreover, thinking is dangerous, because it seeks to question and to get to the bottom of things. It is not permitted for anyone to discover the real truth of things here, such as the ancient understanding of Tao, the purpose of life, the recognition of the worth of individual living between heaven and earth as once comprehended in the older China. Now, it is not the thinking, living individual who is important, but, for the Communist Party, the masses and the collective. No one hits upon the idea, however, that the masses are made up of individuals who, consequently, as individuals, provide the essential reason for all thought and for every intrinsically worthwhile activity.

It is for this reason that in this society the artist as someone with a creative identity has become extinct. The imaginative element is completely lacking, at least in the presentation of China's public image, and as a consequence, the People's Republic has no culture any more. The anonymous masses have driven it into oblivion. Ugly, tasteless, modern pictorial representations, which are supposed to identify the country, depict only Mao and his comrades, the Long March, the muscular fists of a worker raised high, his everlasting grin mimicked by crowds of inane, delighted, stereotyped faces worshipping the image. It is not only boring, but, from an artistic point of view, it is worthless and idiotic. Anything that deviates from it is not allowed, because it is not 'revolutionary' – apart, that is, from a few classical motifs to be seen on serviettes, plates and teacups. These are regarded as mere wares by those who have no aspirations as far as good taste is concerned – that is to say, by the 'advanced' Chinese who have quite forgotten what culture is.

A Talk With an Old Chinese Physician

Professor Hong Guo-Tai came to see me yesterday evening. I had spoken to him at the College of Chinese Medicine three years ago, but had not reckoned on a visit from him, as he lived about 45 miles away from Shanghai in a village where he was responsible for the training of so-called barefoot doctors. This was a form of punishment for him, since he had been involved in the doings of the Gang of Four, which had its main sector of activity in Shanghai.

He came along with Dr Kang and a French interpreter. He was pleased to see me again. We exchanged a few pleasantries, he thanked me for the books I had sent him from Europe, and then we sat down to drink Hong-Cha, a very pleasant dark red kind of tea. He immediately lit one of the cigarettes I had put out for him. Cakes and pastries and peanuts were available, too, and we began to talk about Chinese medicine. It was a continuation of our discussion begun three years previously.

I had a modern Chinese standard work on the subject of acupuncture with me and had marked certain parts in it for our discussion. Our subject was not confined only to Qi (Ch'i), but was concerned with the concept of ancient Chinese healing in general which, Hong concurred, was quite different from that of modern western medicine. The most important departure was in what was conceived of in Chinese as Bian-Zheng, the concept of differentiating syndrome diagnostics. During our training, this had been aligned with dialectical materialism and referred to as 'dialectical diagnostics'. This was not supported by Professor Hong. 'All effective medicine,' said he, 'should be based on the concept of Yin-Yang.'

Like the elderly clinic's physician Ou-Yang, Hong was born into an earlier generation. He had good manners, and knew how to lead a conversation and also how to steer it. He belonged to a generation which had left a large vacuum behind it. Among the younger generation of doctors, there was no one like him who had received wider, all-round instruction. Schools and universities have simply become impoverished in this respect and there are no private teachers. Most of the better-educated doctors of the older generation who had the chance to do so have long since left for Taiwan, Hong Kong, Singapore or the USA.

As a younger man, Hong was employed in Hong Kong for a time. He was probably impressed by the fact that I had once been there as a young doctor. Without saying as much, he clearly wanted to tell me that we two understood what it was like out there. We spoke English with one another. This the interpreter could not understand. Hong could hold his own as an influential medical man within the college and as a party member belonging to a privileged group in the communist cadre. I knew that some of his patients were senior civil servants and were also people who appreciated his cultivated comportment and his wide knowledge of medicine. He was often in Beijing to treat patients or to take part in negotiations. And now we were sitting together in our hotel. I told him that I was working on a book about Chinese medicine. He remarked that the younger generation had considerable difficulties in understanding old medical texts. Despite this, there were modern renderings in the new script of almost all the important ancient works. However, quite a lot of the original meaning had been lost.

I then took up one of the themes I had selected. Hong listened to me attentively.

'The very first problem is that modern, western doctors are taught to view medicine primarily as an objectification of physiological processes with, perhaps, the one exception of psychotherapy. There is a lack of understanding of nature – that is, nature at large, which surrounds us and which supports us – as well as of individual nature, which is present in every living thing and every human being. In this respect, the old, classical Chinese teachings stemming from the concepts of Tao and the universal interaction of Yin and Yang are much closer to truth and to life.'

'The seond problem,' I went on, 'is the so-called scientific re-working of Chinese medicine. In this, the same methods are used in Chinese medicine as are used in modern western medicine – namely, objectivising, quantifying, measuring and carefully calculating what exactly happens in the human organism when acupuncture is applied to a patient. Is this the right method of application in Chinese medicine?' I asked him. He shrugged his shoulders with an amused smile.

'We'll have to wait and see,' he answered. 'We can't measure everything, of course.' He laughed that typical laugh of embarrassment of the Chinese.

'And what shall we do with that special field which is immeasurable?' I asked.

'What do you mean by "special field"?' Hong enquired, raising his eyebrows.

'Just think of the revolution new physics has brought to modern science and to the world,' I replied. 'New physics, quantum physics declares that matter is not built up by matter. If this is so, the origin of matter is not measurable. The primary phenomenon concerns relation, which comes close to Yin-Yang. Matter is only a secondary result.'

'Do you really believe that?' Hong asked.

'Quantum physics has demonstrated it to the world!' I said and continued, 'At the end of dividing matter into smaller and smaller particles something stays which is closer to the spiritual. It is holistic, open and living. It is potentiality, possibility, eventuality.'

'It might be similar to Shen of Chinese medicine then,' Hong interjected. 'Please, go on with your account!'

'Accordingly, matter is just the ashes of such potentiality. Basically, there is only spirit, Shen, as you say in the Chinese tradition, but this Shen is petrified, solidified, and the result of this process of petrification or hardening is matter. In the quantum world there is no such thing as matter at all. Matter for quantum physics is an illusive phenomenon, something disguising reality. Matter is only rooted in our human observation. In this view, the so-called objective results of western medicine conceal the full reality of the human being, which has to be understood correctly as a Whole. That is similar to the concept of Chinese medicine as well.'

'Give me an example of that Whole,' Hong requested.

'As I said: Shen.' I wrote the Chinese character 神 on a piece of paper.

His eyes lit up: 'As well as Qi (Ch'i), 氣?'

We had touched upon this topic three years ago, since the concept appears in the first chapter of the *Ling-Shu-Jing* as a basic phenomenon related to carrying out good acupuncture. I wrote Qi, 氣.

'I could tell you quite a lot about it,' Hong said.

Dr Kang nodded in confirmation of this and added, 'Professor Hong gives a wonderful lecture on this subject. Only our advanced students can understand it.'

'Please speak French with one another,' the interpreter chipped in, 'I can't understand English!'

Dr Kang said, 'Professor Hong and I know English, but not French.'

The interpreter was confused. Apparently, he was to submit a precise report of the proceedings to the Revolutionary Committee, and now found that he couldn't understand what had been said at all. How embarrassing!

'We understand each other very well,' I said to the interpreter in French. 'That's the most important issue, after all. Our exchanges were concerned with the desired goal – that of international understanding.'

The interpreter shook his head and looked unhappy about this. 'No,' he said in a small voice. We had used an opportunity to trick him and he now realised this. Then he took a number of photos so that everyone could remember the occasion and, in so doing, we allowed the interpreter not to completely lose face. We had him translate a few unimportant sentences in French which were quite trivial as far the substance of our conversation was concerned. I knew that both doctors would gladly visit Germany, and I had wordlessly given them to understand that I would one day invite them. That was enough.

At the end of our conversation, I wanted to give Professor Hong a small present, something that I had brought with me from Germany. At first he did not want to accept it, since the interpreter noticed every movement of our hands. However, when we had finished and were leaving the room, I was able to slip the gift into his hand, as the interpreter had hurried on before to call the lift.

In the corridor, Professor Hong secretly slipped a note into my hand. I read this when I had returned to the room. The text was written in English and said: 'See me next Sunday morning at 11 a.m. at the College of Chinese Medicine. I'll wait for you.'

This seemed daring. What had he in mind?

Successful Needle Analgesia

This morning in the clinic a patient arrived with a brain tumour. There was to be a craniotomy during which the tumour was to be removed with the assistance of needle analgesia. The patient had complained of increasing headache, feelings of numbness in the arms and disturbances in moving his hands and feet. The diagnosis was arrived at with the help of X-ray diagnostics and a contrastive presentation of the arteries in the brain. It was an interesting operation, which lasted about two and a half hours. Preparations for the analgesia had been made on the patient about two or three days before the surgery.

We had visited the patient yesterday and the day before in his ward at the Long-Hua Hospital, which is annexed to the College for Chinese Medicine. He was first informed of the diagnosis and then told of the problems of the disease and introduced to the special features of needle anaesthesia. He was acquainted with what would happen during the process. Then the anaesthetists showed him how to relax and how he should breathe during the operation. In other words, a high degree of cooperation was demanded of him.

Yesterday afternoon, his response to the insertion of needles was tested for the last time. Our Chinese colleagues wanted to know exactly what degree of pain they could subject him to during the procedures. The acupuncture sites to be used were intimated to him and were as follows: three needles on the foot on the operative side: Xian-Gu (stomach 43), Tai Chong (liver 3) and foot-Lin-Qi (gall bladder 41). The patient was shown where these points were and needles were inserted by way of an initial test. The patient's reactions were satisfactory.

Four points were used on both sides of the head, namely, Quan-Liao (small intestine 18) in the area of the cheek; Zan-Zhu (bladder 2) passing through the eybrow to the additional point 6 (Yu-Yao) above the eyeball; Shui-Gu (gall bladder 8) above the ear with the needle penetrating underneath the skin until point Han-Yan (gall bladder 4). There was a good response with these sites, which could be determined by stabbing and pinching the scalp after the appearance of the De-Qi.

Yesterday evening, the patient received additional help in terms of pain elimination (in the form of Dolantin) and a tranquilliser. On the morning before the operation, he was given Dolantin again and an injection of curare, a muscle-relaxation fluid.

Chinese needle analgesia is always complemented with chemical pharmaceuticals, something that arouses suspicion among western anaesthetists. 'Which is the actual painkiller?' they ask. 'The medicaments or the needles?'

'Both,' the Chinese declare.

The patient's head had been shaved completely on the previous day. Shortly before the incision was made, the approximate position of the tumour was outlined with Castellani solution on the surface of the skull. It was a tumour on the frontal lobe. The X-rays were there for all of us to see. Both the blood pressure and the pulse rate were controlled and the values noted by the women anaesthetists. These were measured regularly throughout the course of the operation. Both blood pressure and pulse remained astonishingly stable.

Then the operation itself began. The scalp and the pericranium were severed. The trepanation then followed, accompanied by the noise of the bone saw. Below, in the opening of the skull, we could see the pulsating meningeal arteries and the enveloping membranes, the dura mater and, below this, the pia mater. The visible blood vessels were ligatured and the meninges were opened. The tumour now came into view. The patient for his part lay quite still and only moved his eyelids at intervals.

Experience has shown that needle analgesia works best in the head area, using locally placed needles, since the brain then forms its own important substances that eliminate pain – namely, the neurotransmitters, among them endorphins. The brain, by the way, is itself insensitive to pain, so that the patient only felt something when his scalp was cut open, during trepanation of the skull, and when the meninges were separated. He was constantly asked how he felt, and he answered these enquiries clearly.

Very gradually, the tumour was lifted from the surrounding brain tissue, a procedure which required an hour to complete. Small lesions were coagulated with electric thermocautery. After the removal of the tumour, the surgeon asked the patient to cough and to press. In this way, the intracranial pressure was increased to be the same as the blood pressure in the brain's capillaries, something which cannot be accomplished with a patient under total anaesthesia. Some of the smaller blood vessels that had not yet been attended to spurted miniature fountains of blood. The surgeon quickly dealt with these, using thermocautery. All in all, the patient had lost relatively little blood.

After two hours the meninges were closed and the part of the skull that had been removed to facilitate access to the brain was replaced and the scalp sewn together, and after another half hour the operation had been successfully completed. We were impressed.

The day after, we visited the patient in the ward, and although he had a slight headache, he otherwise felt perfectly well.

'It works, then,' Achille announced. 'At least, it worked in this case. What we now need is a sensible theory. Nevertheless, our problem is allowing it to be used clinically in the West. We can't work as carefully and slowly as Chinese surgeons do. At our place, the emphasis is always on speed, otherwise the financial side of surgery would just collapse. At the rate we go, needle analgesia wouldn't pay off, and the patient couldn't hold out. What we need is a full anaesthetic.'

Adrienne, the Dutch anaesthetist and the French specialists shared this view.

In the evening, Achille and I talked at length about this spectacular brain operation.

A Shot in the Back of the Neck

'The brain is quite insensitive to pain,' Achille repeated on returning to our apartment. 'I spent some time in the neurosurgical department during specialist training, and have carried out a few brain operations, so I've tested the procedure myself. Today's experience was quite convincing. Previously, I would never have believed it.'

'I've not got that far,' I replied.

'I've also concerned myself with various means of killing,' he continued. 'Every murder, after all, has its medical aspect. I've had the chance of rescuing murder and suicide victims.'

'Tell me about that!' I said, full of curiosity.

'The best method to kill someone is to shoot him in the back of the neck.'

'Can you explain that to me?' I asked.

'Well, if you really want to know, yes. The background goes back in history. Mao Tse-tung adopted this infallible technique from Stalin, who got his excellent surgeons and physiologists to show him how it was done, since these folks were as good at killing as they were at maintaining human life. It all began under the Russian tsars. At that time, there was medical treatment for the privileged, and this in every respect. You've heard of the research carried out by people like Pavlov, Babinsky, Korssakov, of course. Well, Stalin used their scientific medical conclusions to promote and sustain his KGB, his gulags and his bestial, murderous reign of terror.

'The shot in the back of the neck is ingeniously simple. The victim totally loses control over his body and probably loses consciousness into the bargain – that is to say, from the medical point of view. On measuring his brain currents, he's clinically dead. However, having said that, his inner organs can live for quite a long time and so carry on with their physiological functions in the usual way. This fact has had its commercial advantages for China today.'

I had heard nothing about this.

'After execution in this way, the heart, for example, goes on beating for quite a while,' Achille continued. 'As a result, the inner organs remain intact. Consequently, you can remove them without hurry, deep-freeze them and send them off somewhere for organ transplantation.'

'And you think that kind of thing goes on?'

'Our clinic has had offers of organs for transplantation from China. As a matter of fact, we've never accepted any of them, and that will remain the case in the future.'

Achille went on, 'A bullet in the back of the neck was a boon to Mao, who had learned from his master, Stalin, with whom, by the way, he fell out later. In this manner, he could eradicate about 70 million intelligent, well-educated, cultivated Chinese and so convey them from the warmth of this life to the cold darkness of death.

'In this way, Mao and Stalin offered each other their scraggy hands. Mao, like Stalin and Hitler, wanted to free himself of troublesome intellectuals. They annoyed him, because these people could think for themselves. His followers in China – here, names are almost of no importance – did and still do the same as he did. They just let the job be done. It was so easy: a shot in the back of the neck.'

I knew one thing at least. The reasons people were executed were the same as they have always been: for little lies, which all of us resort to from time to time; for theft resulting from hunger or emergency; for the possession or consumption of drugs; for any kind of stance directed against the regime; for a chance remark; for deviation from the party line in thought or deed; for comments arising from exasperation with the current, unbearable political dispensation; for having ostensible contact with the West, especially with the USA and Britain, as well as for other 'misdemeanours'.

I quoted the wise Lao Zi, who, in chapter 57 of the *Dao De Jing*, explains it:

I took a copy of that book, which I had bought in the bookshop the other day, out of my drawer and showed it to Achille.

'In other words,' I added, 'criminals are created by the state; for the state, after all, has laid down the laws and edicts which are transgressed. For this reason, then, the state is the author of all crime.'

'That's food for thought,' Achille remarked.

'What about a beer to end the evening?'

We descended to the bar, where I tried to pen Lao Zi's characters down on a piece of paper:

法令滋章. 盜賊多有.
Fa Ling Zi Zhang, Dao Zei Duo You.

'The more laws and edicts are known,
the more thieves and robbers there are.'

Chinese Honesty

There was a lot going on the river in front of the hotel this evening. People were standing in long rows along the bank and calling out to others on boats. They were shouting messages or news of some kind with all the breath they could muster. There was constant work taking place on the bridge. Barges overtook one another on the water and boats were so close together that they seemed to push each other.

The room boy came in and brought me 2 maos. That's about 15 euro cents. One mao is 10 fen; a yuan has 10 maos or 100 fen. One yuan is approximately 60 euro cents. We had travelled from the Peace Hotel to our

Dashan Hotel by three-wheeled taxi, which had cost 4 maos – 30 euro cents, that is to say (15 euro cents each). The driver could only give us 4 maos as change for the yuan instead of the necessary 6 maos. So now, smiling all over his face, the room boy was there with his companion, the lift boy, as witness to the transaction, to bring us the missing 2 maos. Thus, the Chinese are past masters in petty honesty. As far as we were concerned, the taxi man could have just as well kept the money as a tip, but there is no such thing as tipping here. That was a dirty habit adopted by depraved capitalists who, as everyone knows, live off the backs of others. That was the way tipping was regarded here in the People's Republic. For us, on the other hand, the trip in an open three-wheeler carriage, so to speak, was much more interesting than the usual route by car. One could watch the life of the city take place at close quarters from an open window, amid a veritable cacophony of hooting, tinkling of bicycle bells, shouting of folks on foot and clattering of the two-stroke taxi engine.

VIII

African Views on Europe and a Farewell Banquet

The only ones who staunchly stood by the Chinese were the African participants. All four of them had become really rather strange. Adnan asked me yesterday, for example, whether we had a traditional form of medicine in Europe. I said that we did at one time, but that this had lost its identity in becoming a part of the medicine practised all over the world. Our traditional medicine was the medicine of the Greeks and of Hippocrates.

To this he replied, 'How come? World medicine is not Europe's achievement; it's the achievement of the whole of humanity. We've all contributed to it, the whites, the blacks, yellow folks and red folks.'

'That is probably what is related in Africa,' Achille piped up. 'You should know that the whole of modern medicine originated in Europe, in France, Holland, Austria, Germany, Italy and England. There was a small contribution from Russia and Scandinavia, but its origins never stemmed from Africa.'

But Adnan would not be moved. 'That's a typical capitalistic lie,' he said.

He was also ready to criticise us because we took photographs, despite the fact that we knew that the Chinese looked askance at this activity. The other day, he had furiously berated Achille for taking pictures, and said that if he were constantly to hang around with a camera slung over his shoulder in his native Cameroon, he, Adnan, would personally see to it that he was shot. So saying, he laughed his deep laugh, showed his yellow gorilla teeth and beat his chest like a drummer. In addition to these observations, he added that the Chinese were far too nice to tourists when they came to China. It would be better, he said, to lock them all up or at the very least whip them out of the city.

Achille countered this with: 'When someone comes to France and wants to take a few photographs, then why not? And when someone wants to photograph me, Dr Habensack, he is quite at liberty to do so.'

But this did not impress Adnan one bit.

A Very Bad Book Published in Germany

I was off again to the post office with some parcels full of books and accompanied by Fishface. It was quite an experience. In one of the packets was the book by Peyrefitte, *When China Awakes*. There is a picture of Mao Tse-tung on the wrapper, and perhaps because the man had such a large, round head, the neck had been shortened below the chin by the designer during the layout. The post office officials objected to this representation of their leader. Who would dare to truncate the neck of their divine master? A supervisor was called.

'Whose book is this?'

'Mine,' I answered.

Another, more senior supervisor was fetched, a man with an evil expression and red cheeks that seemed to have been polished (I could imagine that he suffered from high blood pressure). He haughtily appeared on the scene in a gold-braided cap and glittering epaulettes. He took up the book with his short fingers and chewed nails and removed it to a neighbouring room. It was an eternity before he returned. His face had become even more sinister. He spoke to Fishface in a loud voice, puffing and panting, his sentences short and military.

Fishface interpreted. The book is a very bad book for the simple reason that our Chairman's head has been cut off. The neck is absent. This was a prize piece of impudence! As an officer within the party, he would like to put me in jail for such an offence, and this would certainly have been the case had I been Chinese, but unfortunately he was dealing with a foreigner. A pity!

I told him gently that the book was a gift from a friend of mine, given to me shortly before my departure for China to help me accustom myself to modern China. There was a dedication inside the cover, which he could read if he wished. I would take it back to the hotel.

'That's not possible!' the official rasped. 'This book is to be confiscated by the party!'

I explained to him that the People's Republic of China is painted in a very favourable light in the book, and that the author had been personally received by Chou En-lai three times in Beijing. It was a very friendly book as far as China was concerned. 'So please return my book to me.'

'No,' the big noise said emphatically, 'the book stays here. I've officially confiscated it.'

I refused to bend to this.

'You can read from the title that the book has been published by a

German publishing house, the renowned house of Rowohlt in Hamburg. Give them a call, if you want to protest. Alternatively, you can give me your name and then I can write to the firm. I can complain in your name and in the name of the People's Republic.'

The prospect was a bit too risky for the fat one. Under no circumstances did he want to be drawn into an international political protest. He therefore returned to my remark about Chou En-lai's meeting the author.

'Is that true what he says about Chou En-lai?' he enquired strictly of Fishface. The latter confirmed the fact, although he could have had no idea of anything about this encounter. He only wanted to help.

The flashy fat man suddenly became quieter in his manner, and even maintained that if this were the case, then it was a high distinction for the author to have been so received. It was indeed a good book. A pity he could not read it himself. He gave the book back to me, which I subsequently took to the hotel.

One of the parcels I had packed could not be sent out of the country because there were a number of Chinese stamps worth about 27 yuan in it. That meant that the total worth of everything I wanted to send off exceeded 50 yuan. This sum is the maximum that may be sent off in one day. So I had to return to the post office again on another day because of this stamp collection.

Again, the same old procedure of filling in forms and emptying and repacking books, accompanied by the same stupid jabber of officials for over two hours! However, it went off better than the first time, since in the meantime we had had some practice in packing and repacking.

In the interim I carried on a conversation with Fishface. He began by touching on the theme of Russia as a possible danger for China and was convinced that Russia was a nefarious country and out to defraud. Then he tried to find out what my opinion of China was, as well as that of my colleagues. I told him quite frankly that China must buck up in terms of its organisation of trivial, everyday matters like that in hand; all this had to run much better. It was hardly possible to do anything without being confronted with some sort of ridiculous red tape or organisational barrier. This was an opportunity to tell him about my experiences with the China Airlines employees who had scrutinised my parcels and suitcases for several hours before I was allowed to check them in for Germany. A situation of this kind, I said, was internationally quite unacceptable. Apart from that, the country's technological development left much to be desired. He agreed at once and shoved a pamphlet in my hand, published by Mao, with the title, 'China's Relations with Other Countries'. In it was the declaration that China should be ready to learn a lot from foreign countries and could profit considerably from this. Its Chairman had drawn up some points highlighting areas in which this could be done: better administration, better organisation, greater effectiveness, a more scientific approach and much more. In reading it, I could find much to justifiy much of my own criticism of the People's Republic.

Fishface was one of the few people allowed to come unaccompanied into our room. Evidently, he enjoyed the greatest confidence on the part of his party colleagues. Achille and I once told him that freedom for the Chinese would only come when everyone here could travel freely and when people were no longer treated like dogs by party comrades and civil authorities. At the present time, the average Chinese, if he happens not to be a party member, is hounded to death.

A Trip to Soochow

We were off to the ancient cultural heritage city of Soochow. We had to get up at 5 a.m. and were driven directly from the hotel to the station. Breakfast was taken in the train. It was hygienically packed in cardboard boxes stamped with the words 'Shanghai Da-Shan' on them, and we received green tea at intervals during the whole of the journey. The boxes contained two double sausage sandwiches and two hard-boiled eggs. Next to this lay a ripe, juicy pear. By around eight we had reached our destination, and we boarded a bus at the station. A French-speaking guide was there to welcome us. We then went to a hotel, the only one open to foreigners. Once there, we were acquainted with the details of the round tour of the city.

First on the agenda was the imposing 'Tiger Pagoda', an interesting edifice outside the town. Our guide begged us not to take photographs without first asking permission. Many Chinese were frightened of being photographed, because they believe that a part of their soul is taken from them, the so-called Hun, an idea also associated with Chinese healing methods concerning the liver. In other words, being photographed was harmful to the liver.

Haubensack asked the interpreter to tell onlookers that their persistent gawking was a pain in the neck for him. It was a darned sight more unpleasant than having part of your liver removed! He suggested that it would be better for the Chinese to visit a zoo if they wanted to peer at exotic animals or, as in our case, Europeans. Perhaps in future it would be possible to erect a zoological garden with foreigners inside – yes, perhaps even with cages, so that the Chinese could goggle to their heart's content as we do at the baboon's blue arse. The interpreter did as he was bidden and a cloud of displeasure passed over the faces of our Chinese bus companions. They closed their eyes even tighter and pressed their lips together, so that they seemed to be thin, white lines devoid of blood. Achille's remarks had annoyed them.

After visiting the pagoda, we went on to admire several gardens and were back at the hotel for lunch. While the others took a nap, I decided to go out alone to look around the gardens and streets. One of our accompanying Chinese guides wanted to hinder me from leaving and placed himself directly in front of me at the hotel entrance, holding out his arms. However, he was not big enough for this job, and his arms were too short to block my exit. Without once looking at him, I managed to slip past him. He didn't dare to follow me, and retreated back into the hotel.

The people here were much more friendly, open and ready to help than those in Shanghai. Many of them greeted me, and even remained standing in order to begin a conversation. It was precisely what our official supervisors wanted to avoid. Here, apparently, there are no organised 'street committees' as there are in Shanghai. Here, one can go into the house yards, a thing which is quite impossible in the other city. Folks here wave you towards them so that you can take a photo of them. There's quite a different atmosphere about the place.

Yes, that was it! The party did not want us to have contact with these friendly people, since, in its view, the Chinese here were too naive and politically undisciplined.

A young woman sat at the roadside suckling a child. She was not at all disturbed by anything, even when I asked her if I might take a photograph of her; laughing, she agreed.

Later, we visited a very beautiful garden. The doors that adorned it were all created in the round style typical of Ming architecture. It was called the 'Garden of the Net Master'. We were to go on to look at horticultural displays. That was all very well, but Achille and I had had quite enough of regimented viewing. We fell behind, and went off into nearby streets to get a view of the city's life. In doing so, we came across a very old bridge situated in a very picturesque part of the city. A throng of people had already attached themselves to us. All of them were very friendly indeed. Children took our hands and wanted to see our cameras. They wanted to know where we came from, and I talked to them in my little Chinese.

'Women Ouzhou lai de,' I said. 'We come from Europe.' A murmur of astonishment rippled through the crowd.

'Tamen ouzhou lai de!' they all all said to each other: 'They're real Europeans!'

I told them that we were at a college in Shanghai in order to study Chinese medicine, and this disclosure received a round of applause. They then wanted to know if Chinese medicine was known at all in Europe. 'Well, it's becoming more and more popular,' I said.

At this, there were all-round nods of appreciation. Then came a fellow on a bike who wanted to know what unit we belonged to, and I told him. 'Shanghai Zhong-yi Xue-Yuan' – the Shanghai College of Chinese Medicine. Clearly, this was a satisfactory enough answer. We didn't even have to show our swim pass, a document that Achille had already drawn out of his pocket.

In looking round, we could see that Soochow was once a great city full of cultural achievement. All the houses had a certain characteristic style. There were splendid portals behind which at one time the well-to-do must have lived. For a time, Soochow was an imperial city and the country's capital, and from 1600 to 1910, the business administrator of the last empress of China lived here in a particularly magnificent villa. The empress was overthrown by a doctor, Sun Ya-tsen, who wanted to set up a democracy along western lines called the Republic of China.

The successor to this democratic government has its seat in Taiwan today. Chiang Kai-shek moved there in 1949 after the communists had gained the upper hand on the mainland. Today, this remarkable palace-cum-villa houses a fine arts factory, and behind it there is a wonderful garden in which a number of houses having large rooms are to be found. I took the opportunity to take several photos of both the houses and the garden. After this private walk, Achille and I strolled slowly back to join our group.

We were shown the most famous factory in China for the manufacture of acupuncture needles – the so-called Soochow needles. We used them in the clinic whenever we could, and they were the finest and best needles to be had anywhere. While here, we were able to watch them being manufactured, beginning with the stage at the foundry, where the best stainless steel was cooled and the needles cut to form and finally polished. These special top-quality needles are not to be found everywhere in China, but every self-respecting doctor using acupuncture techniques wants to use them. For us, these needles were extremely cheap, one needle costing about one euro cent.

I bought a thousand straight away. They were packed in small paper packets, each with a picture on them of the famous doctor, Hua Tuo, who lived during the late Han Dynasty (260–100 BC). This was the physician who carried out a surgical operation using as an anaesthetic a herbal mixture called Ma-Fei-San. He was also the man who invented the five animal exercises after watching the movements of wild animals, and from which Tai-Ji-Quan is derived. About two thousand years ago, he discovered the segmental arrangement of the human organism, after which he laid down the 28 pairs of points underlying needle therapy that correspond to the para-vertebral foramina (points) and that are named after him.

He was executed at the advanced age of eighty by the brutal Prince Tsao-Tsao, who suffered from headaches, because he had suggested trepanning as a cure for his subdural hematoma, an injury to the skull sustained in his case during a war. This cure is valid even today as the only correct course of treatment for this condition. This suspicious lord, a man who constantly feared plots by the doctors against his life, felt it appropriate to murder this famous physician, just in case. Physicians lived on a tightrope in ancient China.

After this visit, we were led into the Friendship Store where, compared with the one in Shanghai, there was only a modest display of articles on show. I went into a small textile shop opposite and purchased seven metres of the finest green silk for very little money as a gift for my wife.

From here, I let the group go on while I visited an old Taoist temple situated behind the Friendship Store. Today, it serves as a library, with publications on display about China's Communist Party, calling itself a 'people's library'. I went in and looked round, thumbing through a few books, ever on the lookout for medical volumes, but there was not enough time for research of this kind.

The four Africans and the two doctors from Laos did not accompany us on this trip to Soochow. When asked why, they said that they objected to the fact of being surrounded by Chinese and to being stared at, and also to being touched by children who immediately looked at their hands after touching them to see if the 'colour had come off'. While this may have been true, it was also possible that they could not put up enough money for the excursion. In this respect, we Europeans have more financial leeway.

The day in Soochow was a most pleasant day for us all. At last we had the opportunity to exercise our limbs and breathe fresh air, a stark contrast to Shanghai which, it is said, houses about 13 million inhabitants. The route by train was also interesting. It went through rice fields, passed many a mud hut and travelled over many a canal on which there were simple boats steered by hand rudder at the back.

One thing I found rather charming was that the Chinese live under one roof with their domestic animals. In Soochow, we discovered many a house where ducks and hens went back and forth through the building and where cats were to be seen relaxing on chairs. It showed how closely bound to nature the Chinese still are. Of course, these creatures make a mess, but that is somehow typical Chinese muck which is to be found everywhere. One can find this natural bond even in Shanghai. I once saw a man walking over a railway bridge with a hen under his arm. He carried it with an unassuming nonchalance, and the hen, too, was quite happy with this arrangement. It was not put off by the traffic, but looked around with interest at the people and vehicles going by on the left and right of it. In the town, it was clear that people owned hens and ducks, and even the goldfish that swam in the many public ponds in parks were plied with bits of cake and bread, although the Chinese had little enough to eat themselves. There was a striking number of birds in the trees and on roofs in the city. On the other hand, there were few dogs. In the winter, dogs were eaten as a delicacy, since it is believed by the Chinese that they provide warmth to the human organism. Only in Soochow did I once see a couple of dogs wandering free near a teahouse.

As a matter of interest, our Persian, Ismail, had apparently appointed himself as an informer to our Chinese supervisor. It could have been that he wanted to make up for his clownish behaviour at the beginning of the course, when he mocked the Chinese doctors and professors. He now regularly reported to the interpreters any critical remarks that we made about China and its medicine during meals. These, of course, were then passed on as the latest hot news to the party committees.

Summer Heat in Shanghai

There was such high humidity here that I felt I would like to change my shirt every fifteen minutes. It was very close and the air was saturated with dampness. The thermometer stood at 39°C, and one could wash and shower as much as one wanted, but nothing helped. Even after the shortest walk outside, the collar of a fresh shirt was black with soot and dust.

As yet, there was no Chinese concept here that equated to 'environmental pollution'. Cars pumped filthy blue clouds of smoke from their exhausts, ships on the river released heavy black clouds of muck from their smoke-stacks, and factory chimneys polluted the surrounding countryside much in the manner of a campfire lit by a horde of prehistoric barbarians. For us, this sticky, hot summer weather was, frankly, a catastrophe.

At six in the morning, the sky was beautifully clear, and we watched the morning mist lift over the harbour. There was the promise of a nice day. We used our cameras and took good pictures in the clinic. But in the afternoon, it began with sudden savagery to rain in torrents, a downpour accompanied by thunder and lightning.

When I went down to the kitchen to order a little Hong Cha, a red-black tea, all the boys were hanging out of the window to watch the rain.

'Xia da yu!' they called out delightedly and pointed to the rain. 'It's raining like hell!'

Clearly, they were more interested in the pelting rain than in anything else. I ordered tea.

No, they said. First we want to watch the rain outside. When it stopped, they would bring the tea to my room. What a gang they were! I went back to my room, and it was almost an hour before it stopped raining. Then the tea came at last.

It is ironic to reflect that it is here, for the first time in China's modern history, that people have completely forgotten what work means. Everywhere else where Chinese live, whether in Hong Kong, Taiwan, Singapore or Indonesia, it is precisely the Chinese who are the busiest people. But here no one does anything in the way of work. Why? Because the party indirectly forbids it and because work just doesn't pay off.

To return for a moment to Chinese bad manners. Wherever I went, I noted that the younger generation was rough, bad mannered and brutal. Whenever I walked into the city, I was kicked, and in bad weather, these young brutes hit at others with their umbrellas. There was never any kind of apology. 'Dui Bu Qi' ('Excuse me please') had more or less died out here. Loutish behaviour was on the day's agenda, and if you wanted to tell someone something, then you trod on his feet or thumped him in the ribs to get his attention. If Dr Kang, for example, wanted to tell me anything at the clinic, he did not use my name, but instead nudged me with his elbow, sometimes so hard that it hurt! This was before he began to speak to me. As a result of this form of communication, I went around with blue contusions of the thorax!

Patients, too, used similar call-up signals to draw attention to themselves. I was at the time treating a woman who had painful hip problems and who thumped me energetically in the chest with her fist when she thought the needle was too strongly applied. It hurt. After having had a go at my side, she made an inarticulate sound, something like 'Er, er, ooih!' It sounded more animal than human, and in Europe would be unthinkable. Here, though, it was rather fine, because it was a genuine proletarian sound.

This kind of thing was not only confined to the younger generation that had passed through the school of communism, but it also applied to the coolies and philistines who have always populated China, and who at one time never crossed the paths of Europeans. Older people, and older doctors, were for the most part quite different. Our old Dr Ou-Yang was always gentle, both in conversation as well as in treating his patients.

It was clear that he always considered what was going on in the minds of his counterparts before talking himself, and undoubtely had the better manners. For all this, he was not taken seriously. Dr Kang, for example, treated him as a servant or even simply ignored him.

Concern for others and for good manners: this is something quite unknown to those brought up as communist progeny. With them, unmitigated brutality speaks first, and the only way to make headway in anything is to resort to loud-mouthed impudence or to make the other look a fool in public. In former times, such behaviour would have been unthinkable.

I found myself having to use the same crude methods in my associations with our interpreter, Xiao Gu. Using politeness would only be thought of as so much bourgeois weakness and insecurity. Only by using implacable scorn and contempt was I finally able to gain a little deference on her part.

It is a crying shame that so many of the good old virtues characteristic of the old China have been thrown to the winds. Thus it is that a subtle thousand-year-old culture has been coarsened and degraded to a crude porridge fit for the communist mob. As a consequence, the ancient and venerable arts of China have given way to the manufacture of trash and kitsch for the masses. The new commercial art is tasteless; a Chinese tailor cannot even produce an elegant suit that will fit properly any more, and sold shirts are wrongly cut; even hotel boys have the most unseemly manners.

Fumbling in the 'Pockets' of a Naked Medical Man ...

Not long ago, I was standing naked in the bathroom when a hotel boy burst in without knocking and threw my washing on the bed. He then tore the bathroom door open, unashamedly looked me up and down and stretched out his hand, shouting again and again, 'Wu Mao!' Naked though I was, he nevertheless wanted his 5 mao and 70 cents.

I tried to explain to him that no one, not even a Chinese, could dig into the pockets of a nude man, but he was unable to understand this. Instead of even trying to comprehend what I was saying, he just stood there, shamelesly gawping at me from top to bottom with his black, button-like eyes. He had probably never seen a nude European in his life before. I grabbed a hand towel, pulled the door to – nearly crushing his head in doing so – and told him to go to the devil through the slightly opened door. At that moment, Achille came to my aid like a knight in shining armour, and, without a word, threw 5 maos at the furious boy. Only then did this young knave leave the room, slamming the door behind him and going off down the corridor, shouting and cursing like the proverbial sailor. From that time on, he would grin at me with an unspeakable mixture of insolence and asininity whenever we encountered one another in the hotel. It was quite likely that he had told everyone he knew of the day he found the German doctor in his birthday suit in the bathroom, adding that the latter had not wanted to submit the 5 maos for washing that were due to him.

The two German speech therapists lodging in the hotel, both true-blue Maoists – in other words, communists – were recognised here as 'experts in the German language'. These two informed me that there are a lot of Chinese in Shanghai who are very weak and not at all healthy – very likely because of inadequate, bad food. A large number of people are constantly ill in Shanghai, and that is the reason why a great many take pills all the time. This is the case despite the fact that millions of them do their daily Ta-Ji-Quan exercises. Children, for example, are very often ill for a long time and for this reason cannot go to school.

Our teachers at the college were all them weak, thin people to a man, and Dr Kang was a good example. Notwithstanding, he had something about him that was brazen, something demonstrative of a strong will and determination. Others, like the poor weakling who outlined the techniques of acupuncture of the head to us, were so weak that they could hardly stand. Dr Chu, who was Achille's teacher, and Dr Gan, who once treated Achille, were both mere skin and bone. After a couple of hours at the clinic, they collapsed, and on measuring their systolic values, they were found to hardly reach 100 mmHg. This, almost certainly, was the direct result of malnutrition. Chinese living here only eat a little rice and green cabbage, and that is simply not enough for a working man.

We felt keenly that we were not properly nourished. All of us were changed in some odd way. Achille was quite convinced that we were being subjected to something taken with our food that diminished our sexual drive. It was pretty certain that we were lacking certain vitamins and other valuable food constituents, such as trace elements and highly nutritious protein. We felt as if our bones were slowly disintegrating. Our immunity to disease had fallen off, so that after a pretty strong bout of influenza, I also discovered that I had contracted a revolting condition of athlete's foot, with bleeding sores between every toe, something I had never suffered from up to this time. My feet were in a terrible state. In addition, I was suffering from lack of sleep and missed the peace at night enjoyed at home, as well as fresh air, good food and the occasional glass of good wine. There was none of that here. This situation has not simply arisen from living in this large city, but was one common to many places in the country and, moreover, something that we western doctors could not quite understand, since neither we nor our western patients usually suffered from these deficiency symptoms. In the West, we had our own kind of stress brought about by heavy traffic and the tensions of our professional lives, but here, people suffered from an inner weakness produced by a lack of adequate nourishment and the added stress of being subjected to the incessant party regimentation.

Our food was getting worse every day. Sometimes we had roasted pigskin set before us or parts of some kind of unidentifiable animal. It all tasted horrible and one wanted to be sick even on seeing it.

Yesterday I ordered rice with crab as I just could not face the usual disgusting muck, but this was not possible because I had no 'paper'. My request was conveniently forgotten or the kitchen personnel were not allowed to prepare the dish. A 'change' in the menu resulted in getting nothing to eat!

Today, it was so appallingly hot in Shanghai that the sweat literally poured off the body. It was now 10.30 p.m., and instead of retiring to bed, the Chinese sat in front of their houses chattering and laughing, the air full of ceaseless Chinese music as raucous voices churned out their perpetual revolutionary stew. It was a kind of hell upon earth.

We lay in bed and sleep evaded us in the oppressive heat as the loud-speakers droned on. We could not understand the Chinese mentality. At five in the morning, this mindless row gradually reached its maximum level to spill over into the long day. We never got more than four or five hours' sleep at any time.

Indicative of the mental make-up of the Chinese is the way they drive. There is no consideration for other road users and drivers steer straight at pedestrians, so that it is expected that people will jump for their lives at the last moment. That's too bad for handicapped people who are incapable of such feats. The gesture, for example, of allowing an older person to cross the road in safety just does not exist here. Anyone having power over a vehicle simply tears off in it, regardless of others. And so it is that at peak times, older people rarely get from one side of the street to the other, and many simply stay at home.

This repulsive driving attitude is especially typical of those who currently have power in the land, the senior party-political functionaries. How can anyone drive a car here if he is not a member of this 'club'? Simple people have no say in any matters. A callous hierarchy systematically makes fools of the people. One of the inhuman methods these functionaries use to demonstrate their power is to hoot brutally when they want to get ahead on the roads. Hooting then does not stop at one or two warnings, but is always to the tune of eight or ten staccato signals in a row. Up to now, I had not seen any kind of major road accident, but this kind of thing was naturally kept away from those of us with a western medical interest.

Our female Dutch colleague, Dr Coningk, mentioned a patient yesterday who had arrived at the clinic for acupuncture treatment from another hospital – namely, the Long-Hua. The diagnosis was Ménière's disease. In taking the history, the two western doctors ascertained that the woman had not had her period for four months, and so concluded that she was pregnant. None of the doctors who had examined her previously had noticed this, although it is routine in classical healing always to ask young patients about the course of their period. Everything she had complained of, such as dizziness, vomiting and ringing in the ears, pointed clearly to a condition of pregnancy. Not one person had realised this in the whole Shanghai university clinic. This, too, was a typical case.

Young Mr Gröber came by in the evening. He told us of the impossible situations prevailing in the medical system. Recently, someone had attempted suicide by throwing himself from the roof of Fu-Dan University. It was over half an hour before a doctor arrived to look at the patient. This doctor had nothing with him, not even the minimum needed in emergency cases. The man died on the university premises a short time later.

Another instance was that of a female student who fell ill in the students' hostel. Half a day passed before a female doctor arrived. This doctor, too, came without the simplest of medical equipment, not even an emergency kit. She looked in and then went away again. No treatment took place. Gröber also went on to say that all Chinese who had ever had anything to do with foreigners were subsequently punished or disadvantaged in the most primitive way. One Chinese who had wanted to visit him was taken away by the eight supervisors of the university's Foreign Students' Committee and thrown into a windowless room, there to be interrogated and brutally beaten. In the process, every morsel of information was squeezed out of him: where had he first met this German student? What had he said to him? How often had he met him? Finally, they told the student that he was never to meet or speak to this foreign student again, and if he did so, he would be removed from the university and never be allowed to study further, and that he would be threatened with other disadvantages.

A French language teacher whom I met in the Friendship Store told me about Chinese mystery mongering when it came to foreigners. No foreigner, for example, must ever know anything about the internal organisation of institutes or facilities. He had been active as a teacher of French now for three years in Fu-Dan University's language department, but knew next to nothing about the faculty's organisation. As a consequence, he could not take part in any decision-making at the institute, and was quite ignorant of what was planned for the future. Instead, he was always confronted with fait accompli situations. This made life rather hard for teachers in Shanghai, but, despite this, he was glad to be here. He had certain important tasks to perform in as much as, while teaching a European language, it was also possible to convey information about western culture to his students.

I can truthfully say that mainland China is afflicted by xenophobia, whatever is said to the contrary. Quietly, the Chinese speak badly about Wai-Guo-Ren (foreigners), and tell their children that the wicked 'Long-Noses' will come and take them away if they don't behave, and I therefore ask whether we have then descended to the level of bogeymen and ogres? However, when the travel groups of old folks arrive in China from America, Europe and Australia, these same children have to put on quite a different face. They will have to sing little songs for the guests and dance for them, clap their little hands and cry, 'Welcome, dear friends from abroad!'

This is the way Chinese children are brought up from early on to adopt a two-faced attitude and so hide their true feelings behind a mask of hypocrisy. The long-nosed pensioners on their trip to China have no idea about the hate instilled in these pretty Chinese children by their elders when, touched by their sweet antics, they look at them with tears in their eyes. How many times did I encounter children here who looked at me with hate or fear in their eyes, simply because I was a long-nosed foreigner, a 'Wai-Guo-Ren'?

Final Examinations

Today, we would have our final examinations at Hua-Dong Hospital, which is annexed to the university clinic. The weather was excellent, as I could see by looking out of the hotel window. That put us all into a better mood for what was to come. It was not too hot in the morning any more. After breakfast, we were driven to the clinic, where there was a general mood of cheerful relaxation. No one was too eager to start and everybody called out: 'Xiu-xi! Xiu-xi!' 'Let's all have a rest first!' The noise from the streets below was considerable, cars and buses hooted and the patients were busily talking to one another. Each one of us received a patient. Dr Kang was in the best of spirits, and laughed all the time. Perhaps he was glad that these western pests with their interminable questions would soon be gone at last. He had already intimated to me that he would never again invite such a group of experienced, critical doctors to China. Everyone had found it just too much of a strain.

We would have to give our patients an interview, make use of the 'dialectical' – that is to say, the differential syndrome diagnosis – as well as choose the correct acupuncture locations. This would partly be conducted in French and partly in Chinese. Much Chinese tea would be consumed on the way.

I had been assigned a patient who was suffering from hyperfunction of the thyroid gland. She had the typical symptoms of this disease: insomnia, a swollen, overhanging goitre, loss of hair, much diarrhoea and raised systolic blood pressure. In western medicine, such a condition is referred to as thyrotoxicosis, a poisoning by an over-production of thyroxin, the thyroid gland's hormone. 'Is it possible to treat this alone with acupuncture?' I asked myself.

I had somehow to implement Bian-Zheng in its Marxist interpretation, the so-called dialectical diagnosis. The pulse was fine and thin, but rapid. The point of the tongue was a brilliant red and the tongue itself white and furred. The patient suffered from an inner heat – and what a heat! The heart raced and was also affected. Why? Because the Yin activity was too weak. What 'Yin' was emanating from what organ? Then I hit upon it. It was a heart-Yin-emptiness with increasing heart fire. From the therapeutic point of view, the patient's yin had to be strengthened and the heart fire extinguished. But how? I mentioned the points I would use. Everything was correct. I began the treatment. The woman was afraid of the needles, so that I had to give her ear acupuncture. However, I asked myself at the same time whether ear acupuncture – for this advanced case, a rather weak type of acupuncture – could be the only therapy.

The next patient was a man with paralysis of the right side of the face. Apparently, it was acute and recent. He could not whistle, and tea ran out of the right side of his mouth. He was unable to close his right eye. According to Chinese medical tradition, this was a disease affecting the lines of the 'meridians', a Jing-Luo-Bing. This was fairly simple; I put needles into the cheek and the forehead attached to a weak electric current stimulation lasting twenty minutes. After this the patient could use his lips normally again and close his eye. He was in better spirits as well.

We toasted our successes with orange juice. The chairman of the street committee came in, beaming all over his face, and said, 'Gan-Bei' – meaning 'Empty your glass.' We all obeyed like good children. A little later, an enormous amount of carbon dioxide had to be discharged from our respective stomachs, and there followed a concert of belching that, above all in the Chinese camp, came from the bottom of our hearts. Everyone felt fine and the whole thing was genuinely Chinese. When this was over, the street committee chairman ceremoniously declared that the three of us, Albert, Claude and I, had passed our examination, which brought jolly applause from all sides.

I then gave a short speech: 'Now we've truly conquered the "Gang of Four" and the time has come for the Chinese doctors to visit us. One of these could be Dr Kang, for example. He could then tell Europeans personally what Chinese medicine and acupuncture are all about. He'd also have an opportunity to put quite firmly in their place a whole horde of western charlatans practising acupuncture wrongly and trying to pull the wool over patients' eyes.'

'A very good suggestion!' the chairman concurred, at the same time pulling a face, not quite knowing whether such a proposal was really in line with party doctrine. He went on, 'Not bad. But first of all we'll have to wait for further developments to take place in China . . .' – whatever that meant.

He then wanted to know whether we had any other suggestions. 'We want to improve the situation in our health services,' he explained. 'Has there been anything in our clinics, for example, which didn't suit you?' The three of us sat still and said nothing. It would be better at this juncture not to allow our hosts to lose face.

Then we said that we would very much like to see Chinese medicine and western medicine brought together in lessons, and pointed out that this, actually, was in line with Chairman Mao's principles. We added that we would also welcome more light shed on the combination of acupuncture with the application of Chinese herbal recipes in the various medical specialist areas. With much shaking of hands, we said goodbye to all those who had worked with us: doctors, sisters, patients and cleaning personnel.

Conversion of a Notorious Doubter

Achille Haubensack miraculously changed during the examination. The night before, he had hectically swatted up material until five in the morning. When, finally, he appeared before his examiners, he told them he did not want to be examined, that the course had been useless as far as he was concerned. Therefore, he would hereby officially revoke his registration and return next year to the institute. Only then would he submit himself to a test. At this, the Chinese were in turmoil and told him this was quite impossible. 'You can't do this; after all, it's only a token examination!' they said.

No, Achille insisted – he would come back at a later date.

I concluded from this remonstration that none of the doctors, professors or patients, having been so shocked by him, would want to see this *bête noire* ever again. Secretly, however, they had great respect for him. He should do his examination, please, they said, and then depart for ever.

Everyone talked and talked, so that finally he was persuaded, much against his will, to take the final examination. He was then confronted with a case which seemed extremely difficult. It concerned a man with lumbago. He hobbled into the room, crying out with pain and hardly able to walk. Perspicuous as he was, Haubensack diagnosed this as a disturbance of the meridians, Jing-Luo-Bing, and then acupunctured exactly the points he himself had experienced when Dr Gan had treated him – plus the Yao-Tui-Dian on the back of the hand – and look and behold, the man left the room free of pain and with his head held high like a youthful god!

There was great applause for this.

His second case was a patient having an asthmatic fit. The man's breathing was full of whistles and bubbles. Achille won hands down in this case, too. After a few minutes, the man left as jubilant as a young lark on a spring morning! It was all quite incredible. Haubensack himself marvelled.

And thus it came to pass that a declared antagonist of Chinese medicine became its enthusiastic supporter. The Chinese, apparently, are even capable of achieving this, but that is neither here nor there. A doubting Saul, Dr Achille Haubensack was struck in the middle of an examination to become a Paul, and thereafter a zealous champion of Chinese needle therapy!

But I could not really leave it at that; I had to tell him. 'You know that the party steers everything in this country,' I said. 'Well, your "patient" was a member of the street committee who had jumped in to play the sick man. You just had to be successful, Achille, because they didn't want you turn up again here next year. They've had enough of you. Above all, and apart from this, they didn't want you to go back to Europe and tell everyone what you think about acupuncture. And this you can't do after your success today.'

You should have seen the good Achille at that moment! His surgeon's eyes blazed. 'Don't you talk badly about acupuncture either! There's something in it, even if we've not discovered everything yet. Now enough!' I was lucky that he didn't curse me as a 'counter-revolutionary'. His triumph in the exam had changed his views completely.

The Law of Correctly Stuck-on Stamps

I was able to send off a few parcels from the hotel today. The advantage of that was that not every page of every book was scrutinised before being 'allowed' out of the country. As I was busy sticking the stamps on the parcels, I was put right by a good woman on the reception desk who admonished me for putting them on wrongly. The lower edge of the stamp was not displayed at the bottom and, in addition, the upper edge was not properly displayed at the top. As a consequence, I was obliged to take all the stamps off the parcels, smear them with adhesive and repaste them correctly. The parcels could not be sent off if this were not done, she said. For us in Europe, this would be a trivial matter, but here it was a kind of state project. Small wonder that this country comes to nothing! If I were to have stayed here longer, I would have gradually become just as imbecile. However, I did not want to remain a day longer than necessary in this land of permanent ineptitude and bloody-mindedness.

I had a discussion on Saturday with Dr Kang and had prepared a list with specialist words and expressions as well as the names of medicaments. I also took the opportunity of asking him about treatment on certain days and at certain seasons, which are called Zi-Wu Liu-Zhu, and also enquired about Ba-Gua, or I-Ging, the *Book of Changes.*

I wanted to know whether these ancient rules were still complied with today. He told me that this was certainly possible, but that doing so would take the doctor an infinitely long time, and that was not possible in modern China. It was necessary to treat as many patients as possible in a short time. Long calculations according to the I-Ging and the times of the day – that is, according to the so-called organ-hour – took just too long. On the other hand, he was convinced that by working with these ancient techniques, good results could be realised in some cases, especially in those where mass acupuncture had failed. Whether there was a scientifically understandable and evaluable justification behind them remained something that China would have to find out for itself.

We then went on to talk about Qi-Gong. He explained to me that the patient who had undergone a lung operation and who had groaned and moaned so loudly had practised Qi-Gong, and that he had been previously drilled in it. That is to say, he had not been groaning merely because of his post-operative pain, but was doing so because, as a result of his efforts at Qi-Gong, he had filled his lungs much more fully during the operation. I told him that I occasionally did breathing exercises back home, and asked him whether he had ever practised Qi-Gong. Yes, he said, he had indeed, and not only that, but also some yoga. At the moment, however, he felt himself to be too short of time to practise these things, what with his commitments at the institute, in the clinic and so on. I told him that I felt that the combination of acupuncture and breathing exercises, together with gymnastics, was rather important and said that I had carried out such combinations with patients, and that these had produced good results. He confirmed my view.

'People here in China do quite a lot to preserve their health,' he said. 'Many reach an advanced age while maintaining a high degree of good health. Others, though, often become very ill while still young.'

He went on to tell me of a teacher of his who once instructed him in acupuncture, and who had worked in the tuberculosis clinic until his eightieth year. He walked two hours every day to and from work. He was only able to do this because he had treated himself every day with moxabustion and used a needle at Zu-San-Li point (stomach 36). This was said to be a very important point for lengthening life. By taking advantage of it, old people acquired incredible strength. If he had even once failed to apply the technique, he would not have felt so well. You can see from this that some of the old tradition is still alive. These experiences are not to be found in books, but are passed on by word of mouth.

I told Dr Kang that I, too, felt a strong De-Qi wave when I did certain yoga exercises. He confirmed this. Then I showed him a particular exercise in which I bent backwards and placed my hands on the floor. He thought that I would fall over, but this did not happen.

I accompanied him for a little way to the bus stop. En route, I asked about the Gang of Four. Was it all as bad as it was painted? Yes, he said. Research and the work of intellectuals had been seriously impaired by their doings. I would not be able to imagine how bad it was. The very fact that we could walk together to the bus like this was proof enough of the success of the struggle against the gang. At one time, spies and tell-tales would never have been far away. The fact, too, that we could walk along the river and in the park together and so carry on a confidential conversation was another instance of having won the battle against the Gang of Four.

It was especially here in Shanghai that the Gang of Four had established their bastion of power, filling the most important administrative positions. One of these at that time was that of the city mayor, who had since been removed. Shanghai was the gang's base and springboard, and because of this, the city was the worst hit part of the country.

Dr Kang went into the Friendhsip Store with me. While there, I bought a pair of silk pyjamas. Then we drank an orange juice together. I asked him what he did with himself on his free days. 'Well,' he said, 'I always have a lot to do.' He was free on Sundays, and on this day he would go on a walk in the park with his sons or visit the zoo, find recreation of some kind or play with the lads.

The heat here was getting worse. The temperature was 40°C and we were all nervous and on edge. Everybody wanted to swim, but no one could (or would) suggest where we could go.

There was one other community to be visited, and this we saw on Sunday morning. The visit went off happily enough. I took some photographs. The community in question was based around a vineyard combining plantations for apples and pears with the cultivation of tomatoes. One or two cows wandered around. It was frightfully hot the whole time, and we all received large straw sun hats to protect against heat stroke. During our circular tour, we came across an artificial lake with a small temple on its banks. One or two women were waiting with fruits for us at an open place in front of it. All of us were in a very good mood, and we joked and laughed with one another. I took a picture of our colleague Parviz Fudaghat, the Persian, with a large tomato on his head, and one of the fat Professor Xiong, who sweated profusely as he continuously fanned himself.

In the afternoon I tried to translate some material I had with me, but it was far too hot to do anything. I had sweated through three shirts already today. Although the ventilator whirred and hummed all the time, it was never cool enough. We drank one orange juice after the other and ate ice cream. Fishface came along and treated us as old friends. He thought that I was particularly astute politically speaking, which I am not.

In the evening, he and I went out with a large suitcase to buy Chinese medicaments. With Adnan's help, I had already managed to pack a hundred different kinds of Chinese herbs, so that we could continue to study them at home. I wanted to buy a wall illustration too, showing the famous 'Devil Eater', a legendary Chinese figure who was once said to be able to eat and swallow monsters and evil spirits. This mythological person is still quite popular here, although the communists no longer believe in such fairy-tale figures.

It was difficult to retrieve my passport from the supervisors – that is to say, from 'Old Lu'. Our passports had been taken away from us on our arrival, but for the purchase of larger wares and the sale of my cycle, a passport was necessary. I really would have liked to take my fine, sturdy bicycle back home with me to Germany, but the export of such articles from the mainland was strictly forbidden. Even when I wanted to withdraw the rest of my money from the Bank of China, I needed a passport. Our passports were now in the hands of the police. They needed them to be able to stamp our passports on leaving, but this, like everything else in China, needed lots and lots of time. Lost time!

On Sunday evening, I invited all my colleagues from the clinic to dinner in Nanjing Road: Doctors Kang, Ou-Yang and Gan, as well as the interpreter Xiao Gu. It was to be our last meal together, although there had to be various farewell meals, because eating is the Chinese' favourite occupation. I had at last received permission to have this particular farewell meal after conducting long diplomatic discussions to make it possible. I had said to the Revolutionary Committee, 'Surely a dinner together must be possible, having worked for such a long time together with friends?'

But that was not to their liking. They feared that a lot of party secrets would be given away.

To this, I said, 'But it's a well-established Chinese tradition to give a farewell party.'

They countered this proposal by saying, 'Yes, but we have a restaurant in the hotel upstairs, where you have already had a banquet of sorts. That should have been enough.'

'No,' I returned, 'we would each like to invite one or two particular teachers.'

The two Swiss had already been allowed to do this for their own teachers, so I immediately followed suit and received permission myself. The two French people also were allowed to do the same thing, and Achille hitched himself onto the two men from Cameroon.

The ensuing meal went off very well indeed. We all sat in the same room, stood up to speak and laughed a good deal. Haubensack entertained us with a repertoire of new jokes and, above all, according to an up-to-date Chinese custom, we all energetically criticised one another.

The Chinese turned to me to say, 'You laugh too much and do all kinds of daft things. That looks ill in a medical man. You should behave with seriousness and dignity; that behoves a physican.'

'I don't want to be like that,' I said. 'I'm an old Taoist, that's what I am.'

They all twisted with laughter at this. I didn't want to be shoved into one of their pre-fabricated patterns.

After one or two beers, I began to speak Chinese with old Ou-Yang, and things went very well. Now and again, Xiao Gu stuck her oar into the conversation and said to the already somewhat tiddly Ou-Yang, 'Hey, now stop it! You mustn't say such things!'

But we didn't care a damn about what she said we could or couldn't do, and chattered on pleasantly like a couple of Chinese who had been friends for years.

Albert and Claude had a long conversation with Dr Kang at the next table. Albert had once worked in Britain and his English was good, but Claude, like most Frenchmen, didn't take easily to learning another language. Achille told me that even his French was pretty bad. But however ungifted he might have been in languages, he was apparently a good doctor – at least that's what I had heard in the clinic.

And now something happened that was both odd and sly at the same time. Because it was so hot, all of Shanghai was sitting on the street outside in the evening. The men wore white shirts and played cards. The scene looked like a huge colony of birds sitting near their nests. Given that there were thousands of people in view, it was not difficult to calculate how many there must have been to each residence – easily twenty-five to thirty – and I wondered where they had all suddenly come from. Old grandmothers were hauled out of their corners and placed before the door and children slept there in the arms of their mothers, but at least they were all outside, and they could enjoy the cool of the evening. It was a people's tradition.

I asked Dr Kang whether he liked to sit outside in the evening too, and to this he replied, 'Oh, yes, very much.' Unfortunately, he always had a lot of work, and for this reason he could not often do this, but if he were at home every evening, he would take his little bamboo chair and place it before the door, so that he could talk with his neighbours. It was a pity we couldn't take pictures of this scene, as it was one that was typical of Shanghai's hot, summer evenings when everybody has only one wish, and that is to sit outside and snatch at a little fresh air.

On Monday morning, I got up at five and went for a last bike tour through the town. Nanjing Road was still empty of people, except for a few old folks crossing the street, and I took the opportunity to photo them. Then I cycled on to the park opposite the Peace Hotel and watched a throng of people there. They were practising Tai-Ji-Quan. My next stop was a market where I bought some ginger and a fan that I hoped might provide some cool air. Then off again, arriving back at the hotel in time for breakfast.

We put on our white suits, which now, after much alteration, fitted perfectly at last, and went off to the farewell ceremony that was to be held in the college, and where one representative had to speak on behalf of his or her country. On such occasions, it was customary that we thank our hosts and make a few significant observations.

I spoke for Germany and did so from a sense of pure irony, in that I spoke of the 'Gang of Four', saying that now this criminal association had been vanquished once and for all. The way was therefore clear for an unhindered exchange of experience between Chinese and western medical sciences. Contacts such as these were clearly desirable and were urgently needed, both in the interests of Europe as well as for Chinese doctors seeking new horizons. 'China,' I said, 'must give up the habit of looking inward. No one understands such an attitude.'

After that, we all received our diplomas. The atmosphere was a ceremonious one, but cordial. There were handshakes between us and various city dignitaries, personalities associated with the college, and members of the Communist Party. All of them sealed our new status as acupuncturists having qualified in the People's Republic of China.

This concluded, a large group photograph was taken of us standing in front of the college entrance.

The new academy building was still not quite ready, and the building workers still sat around on the ground next to their bamboo scaffolding that tilted in the wind, as they had done on the day of our arrival. They grinned at passers-by and shouted 'Chi-Fan', or simply took advantage of 'Xiu-Xi' (the opportunity to rest).

It was 40°C in the sun and we were sweating like pigs. Yesterday, I changed four times, and it was 37°C in the hotel room!

A Farewell Banquet

In the afternoon we had a small discussion and then viewed the film that the Shanghai TV company had made on our work in the last three and a half months. In the evening there was a banquet, during which a party member held a speech. The speaker was the most senior representative of the city council and held a minister's rank, but I have since forgotten his name. He was yet another who went on and on about the 'Gang of Four' whom we, as western doctors, had come to understand very well, he said. This alone, he continued, had been a great advance for socialist China. He made no mention of our medical concerns, our profession as doctors or our tasks and activities in the West.

During all of this, Dr Kang surreptitiously looked over towards me. He was thanking me in this way for our critical attitudes towards China's policies, which had evidently helped our Chinese colleagues.

The 'Gang of Four' here stood in general for the Cultural Revolution. In criticising this 'gang', many an unpleasant memory that was still in the minds of those who had experienced it could be compensated for and, they hoped, alleviated. It is devoutly to be wished that this was indeed the case.

While we in our speeches mentioned in no uncertain terms the necessity of liberalising Chinese medicine and, in particular, the Chinese people, we nevertheless received assenting nods from the older generation of Chinese colleagues.

Members of the younger generation, who owed their professional successes to affiliation with the party, were less inclined to concur with this, and maintained faces of stone. Dr Ou-Yang sat to my left and several times squeezed my hand in agreement with what was being said and, in this respect, to signalise his accord. To my right sat Fishface, who precisely controlled our conversations with an iron mask for a face.

Corpulent Dr Xiong, who had singled me out this evening for special attention, filled up my glass again and again, and compelled me to imbibe with his threatening 'Gan-Bei' ('Empty your glass!'). It was clear that he wanted to get me drunk on that appalling 'rotgut', Mao-tai, so that he could get his revenge for all the provocative remarks I had made. As a general rule, Chinese do not carry their liquor too well, and many an institute and public authority has its 'professional drinkers' whose job it is to drink foreign guests under the table when this is thought to be necessary. This large, strong, robust south Chinese individual was undoubtedly the college 'professional' acting in that capacity on this occasion. He downed twenty Mao-tais, which made little difference to his general demeanour. Again and again he let his glass be filled up and shoved it towards me, at the same time calling over: 'Mao-tai Gan-Bei!'

There was no side-stepping his invitations. Mao-tai was always to be drunk to the dregs immediately. Gradually, this constant plying me with drink was having its effect. Suddenly, I saw the doubles not only of Dr Xiong, but also of Fishface, Ou-Yang and Dr Kang. This had not happened to me since my student days. But Xiong was not content with that. To help dilute the threat, I poured loads of Lao-Shan mineral water into my glass after each Mai-tai, and this improved my condition for a short time. But despite these measures, I became more and more drunk as time went on. Fishface took time off to tell me rather awkwardly that this Xiong was a man who gladly drank huge quantities of Mao-tai, but I now began to feel very uncomfortable. After all, said Xiong, I had been a good pupil and deserved reward for my efforts. Ha-ha, I thought, and shoved the next glass of schnapps back to him over the table.

The African, Aladin, then held a good speech in which he summed up the events and the problems associated with our course. As a pious Muslim, he had managed to get through the evening without touching a drop of alcohol.

The ageing director of health for Shanghai was present at the dinner in order to acknowledge our efforts to study Chinese medicine. At the age of twelve, he had joined Mao on his long 25,000-kilometre march through the land. He needed to do nothing more. He was now about sixty-five years old, and the Long March had been his life insurance, enabling him and his family to live very well off the state for the rest of their days.

This long-serving communist could sit back and enjoy his easily won laurels in the People's Republic. All he needed to do for his living was to be present. That was all. In this way, he brought a dignified flair to the show, made a few economical gestures and needed little more than this to make his presence felt everywhere. One or two in our group, notably the Africans, received him with enthusiastic clapping.

I thought to myself: 'Is this what a succesful communist looks like? He has the air of a prosperous feudal landowner; he is now a member of the highest caste in the land, the absolute, uncontested, ruling Communist Party. His manner is one of lukewarm friendliness, but at heart, he is a primitive dolt. The party has merely held him up as a demonstration object. He can boast of no personal services to the state at all.'

There was an amusing master of ceremonies at the banquet who recited his announcements in poetic form. In doing so, he bawled across the room almost threateningly, so that everyone laughed.

On this evening, Achille presented us with a farewell performance. He had already planned something unusual in order to let off steam at last. He appeared at the banquet in his Mao uniform, replete with the cap and red star. Even his arrival earned applause from the ranks of older party members. After the meal, he went up to the old communist and shook his hand. The man stood up to receive this acclamation, and Achille laid a hand on his shoulder. The atmosphere was cheerful and relaxed. An interpreter was called to relay his speech to the audience.

'Much honoured comrade!' he began. 'In my youth, I was also a member of the Communist Party – that is, the French Communist Party, and even more exactly, the communists in the Alsatian basin – namely, Strasbourg. We fought against the Nazis, against an iniquitous Germany under Hitler's rule. So, for this reason, I can well understand the significance of your life's work from personal experience. I would almost give my own life to have experienced what you, esteemed veteran, had to suffer on that Long March. We in the Plain of Alsace had no such march: we cowered in our trenches and worked as saboteurs or fought as partisans. Today it is a day of pleasure, because I have had the privilege of getting to know you, my brave comrade!'

As soon as the interpreter had translated this, Achille once again proffered his hand to the distinguished communist, and continued:

'My hero and model, I must admit to having a request. Please say no if this request should appear too personal, or merely dismiss the favour if you wish. I would like for once in my life to follow in your footsteps. As on that far-off occasion with your Chairman Mao on the Long March, I would like to follow you through this hall on a Short March. Allow me to follow you closely, so that I can demonstrate my communist solidarity with you.'

A Promenade of 18 Monkeys

After this had all been translated, the old party member wiped some tears from his eyes. He was clearly moved. The Chinese can be very emotional, and Achille had hit the bull's eye with his words of adulation. There was discreet applause from one or two tables. The old one, who, in the meantime, had sat down again, now stood up and took one or two hesitant steps into the room. Achille remained close behind him, and both marched, one following the other, through the whole length of the hall, then turned at the wall and marched back in step towards the table. Their rhythmical footsteps and the measured applause accompanying them spurred them on. There was something hypnotic in the air. Suddenly, Erazay tood up and joined the other two, then Jean-Claude Sifferlin and Reto Armbruster followed. Mahmud Atassi, the Syrian professor of anaesthesia, was the next, then Albert Lagarde and Jean-Claude Giroudoux, Adnan Kirinin and Balu. Ten men in all marched in unison through the hall. Initially I remained seated, because I suspected Achille of making a fool of the old man. Like me, the two Dutchwomen were the first to see through this contemptuous charade. They took photos of the ridiculous spectacle, and then bored their eyes into the table, trying desperately hard not to laugh out loud. But when I had got up and started marching together with the group, the two of them, Alice and Adrienne, also rose from their seats, and, still tittering, commenced walking with the others. The two doctors from Chad and the Indonesians had joined in too, following Achille and the Long March veteran with the others, and finally everyone on the acupuncture course solemnly promenaded through the banquet hall. We all turned round at the wall and then walked back to the other end of the dining room. The whole event went on for almost twenty minutes. The Chinese onlookers applauded. We hoped against hope that none of the party bosses present would discover Achille's real intention. But the latter managed with consummate expertise and much charm to bring his Short March to an end and his comrade back to the table in a manner befitting a gentleman guiding his lady back to her seat after a gratifying waltz. Achille bowed several times and murmured another one or two revolutionary phrases. This was without doubt the high point of the evening, and all of us were in the best of moods. The two Dutchwomen, the anaesthetist and the paediatrician had returned to a very good humour and were to be seen laughing merrily. We all sat down again at our former places at the table.

At nine on the dot, it was Xiu-xi time. We all went off to bed. Achille had disappeared without trace. He was not in our room when I came in. His luggage had been removed as well. So I went to bed early.

One day later in the morning we were to fly from Shanghai to Guangzhou (Canton). At eight I was already at breakfast when I discovered some nervousness among the waiters. Half an hour later, there was a huge uproar in the hotel. The local Revolutionary Committee had assembled – not, as it appeared, to wish us a good trip, but to find Achille Haubensack, to interrogate him about the previous evening and, in all probability, to criticise or even to arrest him. The whole night had passed before they understood that the 'memory march' was merely a piece of tomfoolery. They feared loss of face for their honourable comrade and for the College of Chinese Medicine in general.

'Where is Dr Haubensack?' they demanded. 'We have been ordered by the party and the Revolutionary Committee to find and to question him!'

'What for?' I asked them.

'He has tried to make a fool of all serious Chinese participants in the Long March,' they bawled.

'Certainly not,' said I. 'He's one of the most devoted communists I've ever come to meet! He knows the works of Marx, Engels, Lenin and Stalin by heart. He has often quoted them to me!'

'Is that so?' They doubted my words.

'I can swear it to you! Tell you by oath!'

'No swearing and no oaths are permitted in the People's Republic of China!'

This was certainly a lie, I thought, as Dr Kang had told me to the contrary.

With that they walked away, grumbling and mistrusting. We were able to finish our last breakfast together without further trouble.

Back in our room, I discovered that Achille had checked out at nine o'clock the previous evening in order to catch a flight to Beijing today, probably so as to catch an early Air France plane to Paris. I found a note under our apartment door when I came back, saying: 'Hirundo maleficis evolat! (The swallow flies away from the evil!) Have a good time in the paradise of soldiers and workers! Salut! – Achille.'

So much for his words of parting! He had probably spent the night at a hotel somewhere near the airport.

There were one or two pleasant encounters. I had got up at seven in order to secure my bags for the plane trip home. There were difficulties in securing the suitcase lock. I asked the room boy whether he had any string or something similar to tightly tie the thing together. He was just eating when I asked him for this favour, and he appeared in the room still stuffing himself noisily from his plate of rice.

'No,' he said, shaking his head and shovelling more lumps of rice into his mouth. Then, when he had finally finished with his breakfast, he said, bored to death, 'There are shops in the town where you can get the stuff. We haven't got any here.'

I explained to him that I had to board a plane and that I would have to be at the airport in an hour, because we were flying to Canton today. Moreover, wasn't this an international hotel? Surely to God one could find some string somewhere in the place!'

'No,' he said, as he picked his teeth with a small stick. There was nothing of that sort here, and he added: 'You can get everything in Guangzhou.'

I got an interpreter to come over. This person was also our travel guide. I told him of my plight and my consequent need for string, and he said that apparently there was no such thing here. That's how it was here, he added. And left me standing there.

Finally, I was forced to use my belt for the purpose of fastening the case and feared every minute thereafter that my trousers would fall down!

As a farewell trip, we went once more to Mount Wu where, on Sunday mornings – and today was Sunday – old men with bird cages assembled at the top in order to let their birds sing in the open air. Now that was old China at last! As soon as the cage was hung up, the cover on its top was removed and the birdies, which looked rather like tired blackbirds, all began to sing melodiously.

Young lads ran between the cages hanging on the trees, and, with long rods equipped with plastic bags, picked off what looked like grasshoppers. They were in fact large cicadas that caused an incessant row during the night. These insects are pretty large, about three to four centimetres long, thick and fat. They are prized by the Chinese as a medicament to be employed against hoarseness or loss of the voice, because they themselves have such stentorian 'voices', and they are also used as an ingredient in Chinese medicinal prescriptions.

The boys grabbed the cicadas, packed them into their bag and then took them home to feed to their hens, geese and ducks. The other evening, I discovered one of these noisy fellows in my trouser pocket after a walk in the dark. Somehow, he had managed to fly in there. In the evening, he whirred out of his hiding place and sat for a time in a corner, chirping for all he was worth. Then everything was suddenly still. I found his remains on the floor in the morning.

A Sunday morning and the Chinese – mainly older people – with their bird cages. That was a beautiful, peaceful picture. It must have been very similar in ancient China. People walked out of doors in the natural beauty of the countryside quite unhindered. They were delighted with the simplest of things – those that are free for everyone to enjoy.

I thought to myself, *Yes – that's it! That's Chinese nature!* I had been seeking it for so long.

Last night at nine sharp, when the party was over, our host, the Shanghai minister, stood up 'on time' – that is to say, at dead on nine o'clock – and placed himself at the door. This was an unequivocal sign for everyone to leave the place and, on going through the door, to briefly give their host their hand. This was an old Chinese custom. In this way, the guest always gets home in plenty of time after a Chinese dinner.

As for us, we stood for some while on the balcony of Da-Shan Hotel and looked over the illuminated city. We can't go to bed at this hour! 'Let's all go over to the Seaman's Club,' we said. The Chinese declined.

But Alice, on other occasions so shy, took Lao-Li under the arm, saying, 'Now, come on, let's all have a nice time together!'

Dr Kang and Dr Ou-Yang were with us, and old Li yielded to persuasion, much to our amazement. These Chinese would never again see such a crowd of mad western doctors as long as they lived. Even Xiao Gu came along, not so much for pleasure as to spy on us, probably.

Today, we set off in a very hot train for Hangzou. We found something to eat in the dining car, and Albert Lagarde, the professor of anaesthetics, the Swiss Reto and I all fell into conversation. I managed to catch up on some sleep and eventually we reached our destination, with the temperature at 40°C. Thank God there was air conditioning at the hotel, so that at least we would be able sleep at night. The hotel was the only one in the town in which foreigners are allowed to stay, by the way. It was possible that the other hotels had no built-in bugging apparatus to listen in on their guests. After lunch, I decided to stay in the hotel and rest a little in order to gather strength, as I had felt completely exhausted for the last weeks.

On the following day we flew to Guangzhou, from where most of our group took their respective planes to fly back home.

IX

In Hong Kong

Originally I had planned to stay in Hong Kong for a while in order to meet old friends. But when I had passed through customs I suddenly felt very tired. Adrienne Coningk had travelled with me from Guangzhou to the colony. All the others of our group immediately took their flights home from Canton. I planned to stay at the Penisula Hotel, and when Adrienne asked me to recommend a decent lodging, I suggested my abode. The hotel manager knew me from earlier times and I made sure Adrienne was given a decent room.

'Do you have friends in Hong Kong?' I enquired.

'Not one,' she replied. 'But I want to visit the city and get a personal view of the colony and the people living there. Hong Kong is a part of the British Commonwealth, my mother's home country, England. She was born in Liverpool and she suggested to me I should visit it at least once in my lifetime. Do you have friends in Hong Kong?'

'Many. I worked there once for almost a year.'

'Would you like to meet them again?'

'I'm feeling dog-tired. So probably not,' I said. 'But we should enjoy a cup of tea together later in the day.'

'Good idea,' she said.

I unpacked my things and took a long snooze.

An Unexpected Valediction

Some hours later I rang Adrienne. She soon appeared. She had put on an elegant long dress. I ordered tea and crackers for us and we sat down for a chat.

'I've to tell you something, Adrienne,' I began. 'I feel deeply changed after our time in Shanghai. Achille told me the same, by the way. That's why he went back home early. I have the suspicion that our Chinese friends put something into our food. I lost my erotic desire in Shanghai completely.'

Adrienne snickered and shook her head. Obviously she didn't believe me, and even found my revelation funny. After coffee had been brought and we had our first sip, she looked at me, saying, 'Perhaps you should give it a try, Ralf, just as a medical person, I mean, and merely in a scientific way, you know. I mean, you could try it out for yourself to be on the safe side before you go home.'

'What should I try out then?' I asked.

'Whether you've been poisoned or not. It's quite simple, and I think it could well be that you have. You know that soda or bromide are libido killers. Such chemicals are easily muddled up and put into soups and dishes for the hotel guests. If this is done regularly, a male will lose his sexual appetite completely.'

'How can you prove it?'

'Get undressed and let me have a look.'

I was hesitating.

'Come on then, Ralf, get out of your pants,' she suggested, and now I just had to comply. My penis was limp and small, and I felt miserable.

'Come a bit closer,' she suggested.

I complied with her invitation and she tried different techniques on me in order to get me aroused, but with no success.

'I've never experienced such misery before,' I muttered.

Then she said, 'We've had an exhausting journey, Ralf. Let's try again tomorrow.'

I got dressed and ordered a bottle of red wine from reception.

'Tomorrow you might like to show me Hong Kong a bit,' Adrienne suggested as she kissed me good night later.

And that's what we did. We went to the Adventist Clinic where I had once worked as a house surgeon and we met some of my former colleagues. Then we took a cab to Aberdeen and enjoyed a swim at Repulse Bay. For dinner we were back at the Peninsula.

After our meal Adrienne declared, 'It's therapy time now, Ralf. Let's go to your room – I'll give you an acupuncture treatment there.'

When we were in my room, she said, 'Why have we studied it at all for such a long and hard time?' She had brought her needles and some moxibustion sticks with her. I was to lie on my back, and she took my pulse and inspected my tongue.

'What's your Chinese diagnosis then?' I enquired.

'You suffer from a weak kidney Yang, my friend,' she said. 'I'll treat your front side later but first your back.'

The chosen points were well known to me. I soon felt very good. After my back had been treated she needled the front side. She then applied moxibustion on the Qi-Hai point below my navel. Again I experienced a pleasant sensation in my whole body.

'It sure does me a hell of a lot of good,' I said. 'Please treat me like this again tomorrow, Adrienne!' I then asked her. She gave me acupuncture from that day on.

On the fourth day we were walking together in Hong Kong's City Park when I suddenly felt aroused. I told Adrienne, and we returned to my room, where I felt a completely different man.

'You're a miracle worker, Adrienne,' I marvelled. She laughed waggishly.

'We studied acupuncture in Shanghai for a particular reason,' she reminded me.

We stayed at the Peninsula for a full week. I introduced her to some more of my old Hong Kong friends, and then I booked my flight back to Europe.

I arrived in Geneva on 30 July 1978. My wife met me at the airport together with our two sons. They were very happy to see their father again after his four months of absence from home.

'There are many patients waiting for you,' she said, looking at me. 'You've lost weight, darling, and I'll have to feed you very well to get you back to your former weight and to make sure you have enough stamina to work in the clinic!'

X

Back Home at Last

At home I found loads of mail, messages and parcels waiting for me. It would take several weeks to work through it all. On my first day back I received several phone calls from journalists of the local press. They wanted an interview about my experiences in communist China. I told them that I was still too tired to give a report about what had happened to me in the Middle Kingdom.

Achille Haubensack called me on my first evening back. 'I'll organise a meeting with our European colleagues who were with us in China,' he said. 'We'll need a common line about what to tell the European press vultures.'

We agreed to meet two weeks later on a weekend in Zürich. Achille and myself, our Swiss colleagues Claude Sifferlin and Reto Armbruster, the Frenchmen Albert Lagarde and Jean-Claude Girodoux, the two Dutchwomen Adrienne Coningk and Alice Van Anholt and some of our respective spouses and partners attended. We met at the Savoy Hotel. First, we looked at our photos taken in China, and we felt a bit nostalgic about our time there. The wives of the male doctors had assembled in a separate room. They complained that their spouses had come back considerably changed and were less affectionate to them than before.

'I know why this has come to be,' Adrienne explained to them later. 'The Chinese secretly poisoned our meals with anaphrodisiacs that lower the male sex drive. This markedly affected all our male participants. According to occidental regulations it is, in fact, a criminal offence to attack human health, but who can make such a claim against the organisers of our training course in China and the political establishment there? My recommendation as a medical doctor to combat such a temporary dysfunction is to use acupuncture. The disturbances will gradually disappear and full performance will return. Why else did we study acupuncture in China? With acupuncture, the condition will be gone even quicker.'

Surprising Insights

When Adrienne had finished, Achille Haubensack spoke up.

'You know, friends, that now we are back in Europe we are being harassed by press people to give them an account of our experiences in China. We should either decline to do so, or even better, we should paint our time in Shanghai in the most beauriful colours. If we tell them the truth, this will cause international irritation and it would certainly impair our own professional reputation as medical doctors. It would, in addition, not be fair to our Chinese hosts, who did the best they could to teach us and make our stay in China as agreeable as possible. Let us, therefore, come to an agreement today only to give a positive, even an enthusiastic, account to the journalists and to the public. For my part, I will do so. It will be beneficial for our clinics and for European patients, as well as for our Chinese teachers and organisers, who will like to hear it!'

After Achille's initial fierce rejection of Chinese medicine and acupuncture we looked at each other flabbergasted. The two French doctors, Albert Lagarde and Jean-Claude Girodoux, at first disapproved of his suggestion completely. Only Alice Van Anholt and Adrienne Coningk shared Achille's view. But soon Claude Sifferlin, the Swiss surgeon from Lausanne, agreed with him as well, and Reto Armbruster, though somewhat dissatisfied, also sided with him. I thought that Achille's suggestion was wise, friendly and diplomatic. We went into a long discussion about it and then took a vote by which, at the end, we all came to the same conclusion as Achille.

We had invited several journalists to the Savoy Hotel the following Sunday morning, when we gave them a short account. Some days later the major European papers and broadcasting sevices reported in unison: 'First European doctors are satisfied with their four months of acupuncture training in The People's Republic of China.' The full text of our account had been jointly written by the nine of us the night before and passed to the journalists.

When the German press people wanted an interview from me about my experiences in Shanghai and mainland China, I just gave them a copy of our joint report.

Something we could not have foreseen at that time was the amazing success Chinese medicine and acupuncture would have during the following decades, not only in Europe, but worldwide. Professor Hong Guo-Tai had had an idea that he insinuated to me on the occasion of our last meeting:

'We need a new theory for medicine, not only in the West but in China and perhaps worldwide too!' he had said.

I think Hong was surprisingly right and well ahead of his time.

The Great Wall is Penetrated from the Other Side

A number of our acupuncture teachers and Chinese Chen-chiu experts subsequently left mainland China for the West. I had never thought that such a thing could happen. So I was quite astonished when Dr Kang called me one day from Munich some years later. He told me that he had come to Europe with a Chinese study group, but that he didn't want to return to China. He would actually prefer to stay in the West. I had never expected that such a thing could happen and I was thunderstruck. I remembered that Kang was a strictly schooled member of the Chinese Communist Party and had always religiously followed his party's rules. So I asked him what had happened to change his mind so profoundly. He said he would tell me about this later.

Kang asked me whether I was in a position to employ him in my clinic as my medical assistant, or whether I could find him a job somewhere else. I said to him that I would like to think his new situation over, something I did during the following days.

In Shanghai he had seemed to be the obedient follower of Mao Tse-tung's guidelines. We had once viewed a film together about a Chinese woman who was about to become a member of the Communist Party. She had to swear an oath that whatsoever the party required from her would have absolute priority above all other things in her life, even above her family and personal affairs.

I thought of his rather unrefined bedside manner and his harsh tone towards the patients in Shanghai. This would be a real handicap for him in Europe. Moreover, he did not know one word of German, which could be another obstacle as it might put patients off. On the other hand, he had always been quite friendly with me in Shanghai. Therefore, I invited him to see me on one of the following days to discuss matters personally.

'What will happen to your family in China?' I asked him. 'You've got a wife and children in Shanghai.' Kang looked quite gloomy and sad.

'They are in Shanghai, but they will come to stay with me as soon as I've got a job here and perhaps my German citizenship.'

'As a genuine Chinese person, is it your aim to get a German passport?' I asked him. 'I must warn you it might take you years to get it!'

He shrugged his shoulders and mumbled: 'I have no other choice.'

'You have,' said I pensively. 'You could become a professor and one day perhaps the director of the Shanghai College of Chinese Medicine. Just think of Professor Hong Guo-Tai. He seems to be quite happy in the People's Republic, something he once insinuated to me.'

But Kang disagreed: 'He's not at all happy there. He's just to put up with the party lines. And the Chinese have treated him badly as a former member of the Si Ren Deng, the Gang of Four.'

After a long discussion, I took him out to dinner at a local Chinese restaurant and then he stayed with me as my guest for some weeks. On one occasion, I asked him whether he had cancelled his memberhip of the Chinese Communist Party.

'That's impossible', he replied.

'So you are still a member and obliged to follow their rules?'

He said nothing.

He would probably remain a member of that political organisation for the rest of his life! Could such a man be a reliable partner in a medical clinic?

I brought him into contact with Adrienne Coningk, who remembered him quite well from the Shanghai College times. She came over to meet him and agreed to employ him at her clinic in Groningen, so he went back with her to the Netherlands. Later he went to work in a pain clinic in Amsterdam, where he still is. He managed to get permission from the Netherlands authorities and the Chinese government for his wife and children to visit him in Amsterdam, and they, of course, did not want to go back to Shanghai either, but wanted to stay with him in Amsterdam.

About a year later, Professor Hong Guo-Tai unexpectedly phoned me from London, where he was attending a conference. I invited him to come and see me, and I sent him a train ticket to Germany. After he arrived, he informed me that he had the same intention as Dr Kang: he did not want to go back to China. He lived with me for a couple of months and we thoroughly discussed all aspects of Chinese medicine, as well as the pros and cons of a physician's professional life in both China and Europe. I did not want to employ him for the same reasons I had not wanted to emply Kang. First of all, he was a medical celebrity. One day, however, I found the opportunity for him to work in a clinic in San Francisco. He went there, and he still lives there together with his wife, who was miraculously permitted to leave China.

Both Kang and Hong spread the information that I had assisted them in the business of leaving the People's Republic of China and finding a job in the West. Consequently, I then received a lot of requests from other Chinese physicians or their European friends who asked me for the same support.

Occasionally, I consulted Achille Haubensack about this problem. He was by then running a successful Chen-chiu clinic in Nancy in addition to his work as a surgeon. He invited me to visit him in Nancy from time to time.

Once when we met, he said to me, 'You, Ralf, and I, we've done something for the sake of Chinese medicine and acupuncture in Europe, haven't we?' And he went on to advocate my view completely. 'We have both become quite popular as "Chinese doctors" in western countries. If we get more and more Chinese doctors coming here from abroad, from mainland China, doing the same thing as us – where will that leave us in the future?'

'As experienced medical men, we understand more of western medicine than our Chinese immigrant colleagues do', I pointed out.

'That's an advantage,' Achille agreed.

'*Hirundo maleficis evolat*! [The swallow flies away from the evil!]', I recited. 'That's what I've gladly adopted from you!'

He giggled. 'And the maleficent, the evil-doing witchcraft, as far as Chinese medicine and acupuncture goes in the West, is lack of knowledge of western medicine. You see what I mean?'

'I see and I agree! Western medicine should be understood thoroughly beforehand.'

'Ugh! That's a tricky and difficult job,' Achille hissed. 'Have you really understood it, Ralf?'

'I'm not sure, Achille,' I admitted.

We looked at each other and started laughing. We laughed for quite a while.

'I'll tell you something, Ralf: I have only understood western medicine completely after I'd studied Chinese medicine in Shanghai', he said.

'Then we've somehow managed to get through the Great Wall and get back again on our trip there, haven't we?'.

'I hope so, Ralf – I feel quite similar to you,' said Achille.

OH, East is East, and West is West, and never the twain shall meet,
Till Earth and Sky stand presently at God's great Judgment Seat;
But there is neither East nor West, Border, nor Breed, nor Birth,
When two strong men stand face to face, tho' they come from the ends of the earth!